P9-CFA-731

Contents

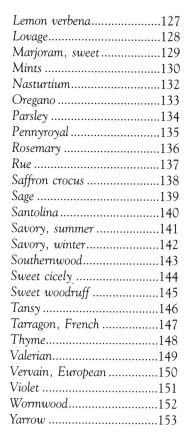
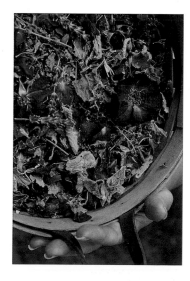

INTRODUCTION

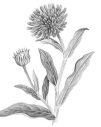

Gardeners everywhere are rediscovering the magic of herbs and herb gardens. Perhaps some of this rekindled interest comes from the increasing awareness of the interaction between good nutrition and good health – nothing makes a meal of whole foods taste more delicious than some well-chosen herbal seasonings. Fine flavor is another good reason. Freshly picked herbs from the backyard garden are a thousand times more flavorful than those from the grocery cooler. Home-dried herbs are also far superior to those that may have been dried a year or two before and left in storage until they were put on the shelf. And where can you get frozen herbs except from your own freezer? For herbs that lose flavor when they are dried, home-frozen supplies are the only way to guarantee that you can season foods in winter with the fresh tastes of summer.

Herbs are easy to grow. If you give them the growing conditions they prefer, most of them will take less care than almost anything else in your garden. If you are a beginning gardener, herbs are a must for you. Not only is their care simple and straightforward, but the results you get will spur you on to greater gardening successes. More advanced gardeners also appreciate herbs' easy-growing nature. Once established, a truly spectacular herb garden will take so little effort to maintain that you will have time to spare for vegetables, fruits, and flowers.

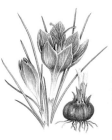

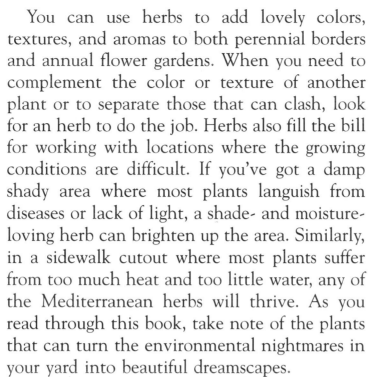

You can use herbs to add lovely colors, textures, and aromas to both perennial borders and annual flower gardens. When you need to complement the color or texture of another plant or to separate those that can clash, look for an herb to do the job. Herbs also fill the bill for working with locations where the growing conditions are difficult. If you've got a damp shady area where most plants languish from diseases or lack of light, a shade- and moisture-loving herb can brighten up the area. Similarly, in a sidewalk cutout where most plants suffer from too much heat and too little water, any of the Mediterranean herbs will thrive. As you read through this book, take note of the plants that can turn the environmental nightmares in your yard into beautiful dreamscapes.

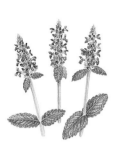

From hair rinses to headache medications, herbal preparations are also coming into vogue again. Not only are these preparations better for you and the environment, they are also very effective. With the right herbs in your garden, for example, you'll never need to buy another box of nasty-smelling mothballs to protect your woolens. The fragrance of a homemade pot-pourri is so much more lovely than its synthetic counterparts that you'll wonder why anyone uses commercial air fresheners.

So go ahead and plant that herb garden. The suggestions in this book, from design to final use, should help you lay the foundation for a beautiful herb garden that adds pleasure to almost every aspect of your life.

Chapter

1

PLANNING AND PREPARING YOUR HERB GARDEN

❧

HERB GARDENS *are a delight in every possible way. They look beautiful. They smell wonderful. And with a bit of planning and preparation, they are relatively care-free. The herbs they produce are also a treat. The fresh flavors of culinary herbs add pizzazz to otherwise mundane meals. And that's only the beginning of the uses you'll find for your herbs. Create your own flavored vinegars and oils. Make delightfully fragrant cosmetics for your skin and hair. Design attractive and aromatic herbal arrangements and potpourris. Or mix up a batch of environmentally friendly, homegrown insect repellent. Just as the herbs you can grow in your garden are marvelously diverse, so are the many ways in which you can use them. In this chapter you'll find everything you need to help you plan an herb garden that pleases your eye and keeps you well supplied with the herbs you use most. Learn how to choose the best site for your herb garden, how to create a formal or more casual look, and even the number of plants you'll need to satisfy your herbal needs throughout the year.*

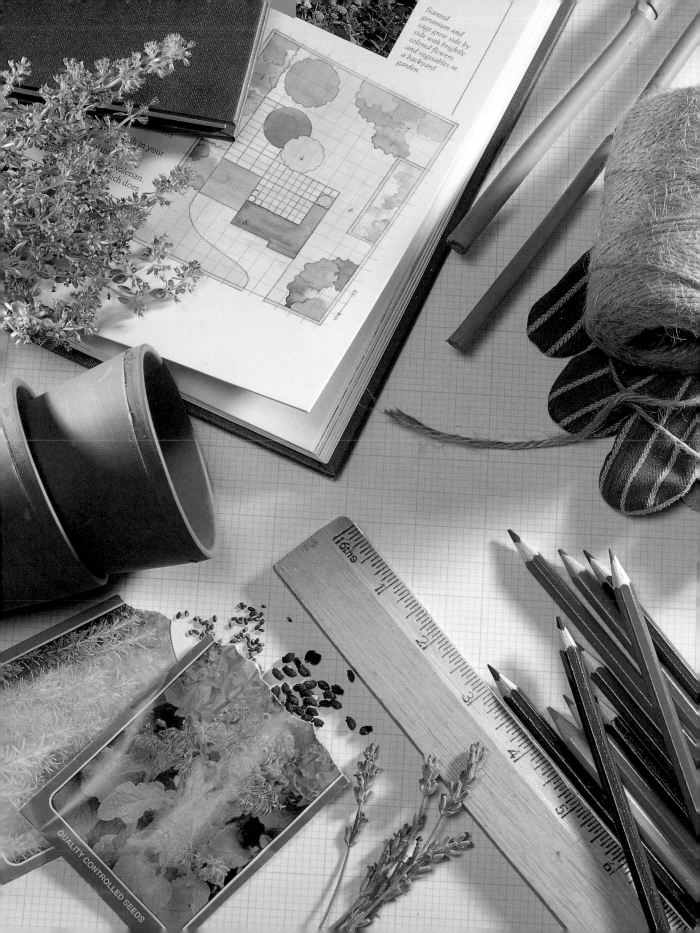

Scented
geranium and
sage grow side by
side with brightly
colored flowers
and vegetables in
a backyard
garden.

Choosing Your Plants

Herb gardens have a special magic. Filled with alluring fragrances, colors, textures, and flavors, they reflect a rich and diverse history. Used to flavor our food, to treat our ailments, and to soothe our souls, herbs enhance our lives in so many ways that it is hard to imagine doing without them.

In the garden, herbs represent both practicality and pleasure. Even the most steadfast vegetable growers make room for a few basil plants for flavoring their tomatoes. And a patch of lavender is a fragrant indulgence that lends its aroma to potpourris and sachets all year long.

When your interest in herbs grows beyond simply tucking in a few plants amid your flowers or vegetables, it's time to celebrate herbs in a garden of their very own. Plan an herb garden that suits your personal tastes, style, and needs. One of the most enjoyable parts of planning your herb garden is choosing the plants you want to grow. The world of herbs is far larger than you may have imagined, as you'll discover the first time you open a catalog from a company that specializes in herbs. (See page 155 for a list of resources.) Some seed companies list as many as 28 types of basil and 21 different thymes! And that's only the beginning.

How many different herbs are there? It's likely no one knows for certain because, as communication and travel open up areas that were once inaccessible, we continue to find more herbs. Some are unknown on the North American continent, while others are newly discovered relatives of familiar favorites. We're also learning to appreciate our own American herbs, used in native medicine long before Columbus crossed the Atlantic. Added to this wealth are the many cultivars of plants we already know and love.

START SMALL

Even if you long to grow all 21 kinds of thyme and all 28 basils, it's wise to start small. No matter whether we're beginning gardeners or veterans, most of us have a tendency to plant more than we can weed. That's why it's a good idea to keep your time budget in mind, as well as your checkbook, when ordering seeds and plants. It's tempting to get carried away while you're planning the garden, but your herbs will give you greater pleasure if they're easy to tend.

CHOOSE WHAT YOU'LL USE

Are you a good cook who uses bunches of fresh herbs during the summer and jars of dry ones in the winter? Maybe you line the shelves with fancy vinegars or oils. Or maybe you routinely make potpourris and herbal wreaths and swags. Whatever your interest, choose the plants appropriate to it.

Start with the basics. If you usually cook with only a handful of basic herbs, grow them before you launch into the ones that require new recipes. If you're interested in making herbal wreaths, begin by growing a limited selection of plants that you know you'll use – mainstays like artemisia and lavender, for example.

But keep in mind that experimenting with new herbs is part of the fun of herb gardening. Be sure to tuck some new-to-you herbs in among the regulars every year. With such a bounty of herbs to choose from, you're bound to meet some new favorites along the way.

HERBS AT A GLANCE

Herb	Life Cycle	Hardy to Zone	Light	Soil	Use
Aloe	Tender perennial; grown as houseplant	10	Partial sun to full sun	Sandy, well drained	Medicinal
Angelica	2–3 years; see Directory, page 101	4	Partial shade to full sun	Moist, slightly acid	Culinary
Anise	Annual		Full sun	Sandy, well drained	Culinary, medicinal
Anise hyssop	Perennial	5	Full sun	Moist, fertile, well drained	Culinary, tea, medicinal; repels imported cabbage moth
Basil, sweet	Annual		Full sun	Moist, fertile	Culinary, ornamental, crafts, medicinal; companion to tomatoes
Bee balm	Perennial; can be invasive	3	Partial shade to full sun	Moist, fertile	Culinary, tea, crafts
Betony	Perennial	4	Filtered shade to partial sun	Moist but well drained	Tea, medicinal, ornamental
Borage	Annual; self-seeds easily		Full sun to partial sun	Moist, fertile, well drained	Culinary, tea; attracts bees
Calendula	Annual		Full sun	Average fertility, well drained	Culinary, medicinal, cosmetic
Caraway	Annual or biennial	3	Full sun to filtered shade	Sandy, fertile, well drained	Culinary, medicinal
Catnip	Perennial	3	Full sun to partial shade	Average fertility, well drained	Tea, medicinal, crafts, cosmetic
Chamomile, German	Annual		Full sun	Well drained	Tea, medicinal, cosmetic
Chamomile, Roman	Perennial	5	Partial shade	Average fertility	Tea, medicinal, cosmetic
Chervil	Annual		Partial to filtered shade	Moist, fertile	Culinary ▷

Chamomile   Calendula   Basil   Borage   Angelica

HERBS AT A GLANCE (Continued)					
Herb	Life Cycle	Hardy to Zone	Light	Soil	Use
Chives	Perennial	3	Full sun	Moist, fertile, well drained	Culinary, ornamental
Cilantro	Annual		Full sun to partial shade	Moist, fertile, well drained	Culinary
Clary	Biennial	4	Full sun	Well drained, average fertility	Culinary, medicinal, ornamental, aromatic, cosmetic
Comfrey	Perennial; can be invasive	3	Full sun to partial shade	Moist, fertile, well drained	Medicinal (for external use only), cosmetic
Dill	Annual; self-seeds easily		Full sun	Moist, fertile, well drained	Culinary; attracts bees and other beneficial insects
Fennel	Perennial, grown as annual	3	Full sun	Moist, fertile, well drained	Culinary, medicinal, ornamental, cosmetic
Feverfew	Perennial	5	Full sun	Average	Ornamental, dried arrangements, medicinal
Geraniums, scented	Perennial (over-winter indoors)	10	Full sun	Moist, fertile, well drained	Ornamental, aromatic for potpourris; feeds beneficials
Hyssop	Perennial	4	Full sun to partial shade	Light, well drained	Culinary, tea, ornamental, cosmetic; attracts bees
Lavender	Perennial	5–8	Full sun	Light, well drained	Aromatic, crafts, ornamental, culinary, cosmetic, medicinal
Lemon balm	Perennial	4	Full sun to partial shade	Average, well drained	Tea, culinary, aromatic, cosmetic; attracts bees

Scented geranium   Chives   Comfrey   Lavender   Fennel

Herb	Life Cycle	Hardy to Zone	Light	Soil	Use
Lemongrass	Perennial (over-winter indoors)	9	Full sun to partial shade	Fertile, deep, moist, well drained	Culinary, tea, aromatic
Lemon verbena	Perennial (over-winter indoors)	9	Full sun	Fertile, deep, moist	Aromatic, tea, culinary, cosmetic
Lovage	Perennial	4	Full sun to partial shade	Fertile, moist, well drained	Culinary, medicinal
Marjoram, sweet	Perennial, grown as annual	10	Full sun	Light, dry, well drained	Culinary, ornamental, crafts
Mints	Perennial	4–5	Full sun to partial shade	Fertile, moist, well drained	Culinary, tea, aromatic, medicinal, cosmetic
Nasturtium	Annual		Full sun to partial shade	Low fertility, moist, well drained	Ornamental, culinary, cosmetic
Oregano	Perennial	5	Full sun	Average, well drained	Culinary, crafts, medicinal
Parsley	Biennial	5	Full sun to partial shade	Fertile, moist, well drained	Culinary, cosmetic
Pennyroyal	Perennial	5	Full sun to partial shade	Fertile, moist, well drained	Cosmetic; insect repellent
Rosemary	Perennial (over-winter indoors)	8	Full sun	Fertile, very well drained	Culinary, aromatic for potpourris, medicinal, cosmetic
Rue	Perennial	4	Full sun	Low fertility, well drained	Ornamental, dried arrangements; insect repellent
Saffron crocus	Perennial	6	Full sun to partial shade	Sandy, well drained	Culinary
Sage	Perennial	4	Full sun to partial shade	Average, well drained	Culinary, medicinal, dried crafts, cosmetic
Santolina	Perennial	6	Full sun	Low fertility, well drained	Dried crafts; insect repellent ▷

Nasturtium   Saffron crocus   Rosemary   Mint   Oregano

HERBS AT A GLANCE (Continued)

Herb	Life Cycle	Hardy to Zone	Light	Soil	Use
Savory, summer	Annual		Full sun	Low fertility, well drained	Culinary
Savory, winter	Perennial	5	Full sun	Low fertility, well drained	Culinary
Southernwood	Perennial	4	Full sun	Average, well drained	Dried crafts, cosmetic; insect repellent
Sweet cicely	Perennial	3	Filtered sun to partial shade	Rich, moist, well drained	Culinary, ornamental
Sweet woodruff	Perennial	3	Shade to partial shade	Moist, humusy, well drained	Aromatic, dried potpourris and herbal wreaths
Tansy	Perennial	4	Full sun to partial shade	Average, well drained	Dried crafts and arrangements; insect repellent
Tarragon, French	Perennial	4	Full sun to partial shade	Average, well drained	Culinary
Thyme	Perennial	5	Full sun to partial shade	Sandy, well drained	Culinary, ornamental, cosmetic; insect repellent
Valerian	Perennial	4	Full sun to partial shade	Rich, moist, well drained	Ornamental, medicinal
Vervain, European	Annual		Full sun	Rich, moist, well drained	Ornamental
Violet	Perennial	5	Partial shade to full sun	Rich, moist, well drained	Ornamental, culinary
Wormwood	Perennial	4	Full sun to partial shade	Low fertility, well drained	Dried crafts; insect repellent
Yarrow	Perennial	2	Full sun	Rich, well drained	Ornamental, dried arrangements, cosmetic

Thyme   Santolina   Violet   Savory   Tansy

Choosing Locations

Location is the secret to growing healthy, luxuriant herbs. Herb plants that grow where soil conditions and light exposure meet their requirements are largely trouble-free. Some herbs like it sunny, hot, and dry, while others thrive in moist soil and filtered sunlight. While you're choosing plants, think about where they'll grow. Check the charts on pages 9–12 to find many common herbs that are right for your site.

W ith a little ingenuity, you can grow plants that at first glance might not be suited to your garden. If your patio is the only consistently sunny spot on your property, for example, you can set out heat-loving herbs in large pots. Or maybe you don't have a speck of shade in the yard. In that case, you might want to think about positioning plants that prefer cool sites to the east of a row of sunflowers and pole beans. The taller plants will cast some welcome shade right where your herbs want it.

SOIL CONDITIONS

Herbs have a reputation for growing best in soils with very low fertility levels, but this is true of only a few of them. Most are healthier and more productive in soils of average fertility, and a few require the rich soils typically found in the vegetable garden. Adding compost to your soil will incorporate some needed nutrients, and it's unlikely to create nutrient imbalances. Aged, well-rotted manure is also excellent for improving soil fertility. Check the "Herbs at a Glance" chart on pages 9–12.

SOIL MOISTURE PREFERENCES OF HERBS

Prefer dry soil:

Aloe	Chives
Anise	Dill
Caraway	Fennel
Chamomile	Lemon verbena
Clary	Saffron crocus
Feverfew	Tansy
Garlic chives	**Prefer moist soil:**
Hyssop	Angelica
Lavender	Basil
Marjoram, sweet	Bee balm
Oregano	Calendula
Rosemary	Catnip
Rue	Chervil
Sage	Cilantro
Santolina	Comfrey
Savory, summer	Geraniums, scented
Savory, winter	Lemon balm
Southernwood	Lemongrass
Tarragon	Lovage
Thyme	Mints
Wormwood	Nasturtium
Prefer moderately	Parsley
moist soil:	Pennyroyal
Anise hyssop	Sweet cicely
Betony	Sweet woodruff
Borage	Valerian
	Violet

Good soil drainage is essential in the herb garden. Even the herbs that require high soil moisture will not tolerate waterlogged soil. Soggy soils favor the growth of microorganisms that cause root diseases. In well-drained soil, roots can withstand heavy rainfall and snow runoff. Increasing the amount of organic matter in your soil by adding compost or organic mulches improves both the drainage and moisture-holding capacity of the soil.

Some soils are wet only seasonally. If your soil

is consistently wet only during the early spring and late fall, you can simply raise the level of the bed by heaping several inches of soil from the pathways onto the bed area. If your soil has severe drainage problems, plant your herbs in double-dug or permanent raised beds. (See "Resources" on page 155 for reference books that describe these procedures.)

HOW MOIST IS MOIST?

In well-drained soils, the time between waterings determines whether a soil is dry, moderately moist, or moist.

Many of our favorite herbs hail from the sandy, rocky soils around the Mediterranean Sea. These plants tend to thrive in loose soils that are deeply but infrequently watered. For plants that prefer dry soils like these, let the top few inches of the soil surface dry between waterings.

Moist soils are those that remain about as damp as a squeezed-out sponge. To give your herbs moist-soil conditions, allow only the top $\frac{1}{2}$ inch of soil to dry out between waterings. However, avoid watering so often that the top is always wet.

Moderately moist soils fall between these two extremes. For herbs that prefer this condition, let an inch or so of surface soil dry between waterings.

LIGHT

The duration and intensity of sunlight falling on your herbs also determine their health. We commonly use the following terms to describe light conditions:

Full sun means that plants receive at least six hours of direct sunlight a day and filtered light for the remaining hours.

Partial shade refers to a site where plants receive at least four hours of direct sunlight a day and filtered sunlight or shade for the remaining time.

Shade describes a situation where plants receive some filtered sunlight for part of the day, generally the morning, but are shaded by a dense

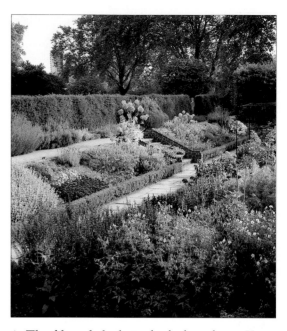

▲ **The filtered shade** *in this herb garden at Kew, England, provides the best environment for each herb growing there. Sun lovers grow in the center, where the light is more intense.*

canopy or wall during the afternoon.

Light is filtered when it travels through a shifting canopy of overhead leaves. Light intensity varies with the time of day. Direct morning light is never as intense as direct light from noon through the afternoon hours. This difference means that a plant that prefers partial shade is more likely to grow well where it receives five hours of direct morning light than with five hours of direct afternoon light.

Often plants can tolerate less than ideal circumstances, especially if you tinker with other factors in their environment. For example, even if you have a site that receives less than six hours a day of direct sunlight, "full sun" plants will prosper if they grow where light is reflected from a smooth, white wall. If you wanted to grow "partial shade" plants in the same spot, you'd be wise to back them up with a dark, rough-textured wall or dense, evergreen hedge.

LIGHT PREFERENCES OF HERBS

Many plants have definite preferences when it comes to sun and shade; they thrive only in the right light. Others will tolerate a wider range of exposures, although they may grow less vigorously than they would if planted in their preferred light conditions.

Prefer shade:
Sweet cicely
Sweet woodruff

Tolerate shade:
Angelica
Chervil
Lemon balm
Lovage
Mints
Parsley
Saffron crocus
Valerian
Violet

Prefer partial shade:
Angelica
Bee balm
Betony
Chervil
Lemon balm
Lovage
Mints
Pennyroyal
Tansy
Valerian

Violet

Tolerate partial shade:
Anise hyssop
Borage
Calendula
Catnip
Chamomile
Chives
Cilantro
Comfrey
Fennel
Feverfew
Hyssop
Marjoram, sweet
Rosemary
Rue
Saffron crocus
Savory, summer
Savory, winter
Sweet cicely
Sweet woodruff
Tarragon
Thyme
Wormwood

Prefer full sun:
Aloe
Anise
Anise hyssop
Basil
Borage
Calendula
Caraway
Catnip
Chamomile
Chives
Cilantro
Clary
Comfrey
Dill
Fennel
Feverfew
Garlic chives
Geraniums, scented
Hyssop
Lavender
Lemon verbena
Marjoram, sweet
Oregano

Parsley
Rosemary
Rue
Saffron crocus
Sage
Santolina
Savory, summer
Savory, winter
Southernwood
Tarragon
Thyme
Wormwood

Tolerate full sun:
Angelica
Bee balm
Betony
Lemon balm
Lovage
Mints
Pennyroyal
Tansy
Valerian
Violet

► **Try** *using these herbs as companions in your vegetable garden.*

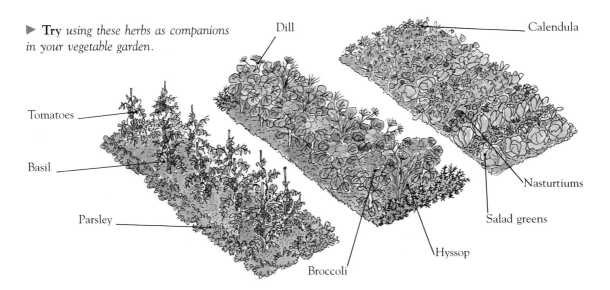

Tomatoes
Basil
Parsley
Dill
Broccoli
Hyssop
Calendula
Nasturtiums
Salad greens

Designing Your Garden

A good design can make your herb garden the most care-free spot in your yard as well as the most beautiful. As you plan, keep both of these goals in mind. It's easier to maintain a garden where every plant is easy to reach than one where plants are inaccessible. It's also much more rewarding to devote a few hours of weeding time to a garden that looks spectacular afterward than to one where you can hardly see the difference.

DESIGNING FOR BEAUTY

Traditionally, herb gardens have been laid out in very formal, geometric patterns such as those on this page. Formal gardens, with their regular and repeating areas and restful blue-green, gray, and silver hues, create a serene atmosphere.

Some contemporary herb gardens, on the other hand, are more free-form and spontaneous in feeling. Rather than adhering to a rigid geometric shape, their curved lines form an irregular outline and the resulting garden layout resembles that of a perennial bed.

Despite the differences between formal and informal styles, they share many elements of good garden design. When planning your herb garden, keep these basic design elements in mind.

Shape: The shape of your herb garden determines much of its character. Both the overall outline – whether it's a circle, rectangle, or teardrop – as well as the shapes within that area, define the form. The human eye tries to simplify what it sees into known shapes. Even when you are planning an informal garden, it will be more pleasing if the interior spaces are somewhat geometric.

Interior spaces are created first by pathways and then by plant groupings. Plan the pathways so that they complement the garden's outline. For example, a simple cross can make a nice pathway in a circular garden but could be out of place in a teardrop-shaped area. Here, curved paths that mirror the outside dimension, with stepping-stones between the paths, may be more appropriate.

Repetition: Repeating form and color unifies a garden, no matter how diverse the plantings. If you are musical, think of repeating elements as the "rhythm" of a garden, and design for the rhythm that makes you feel most comfortable. Even if a score of different herbs are growing in that teardrop-shaped garden, for instance, two or

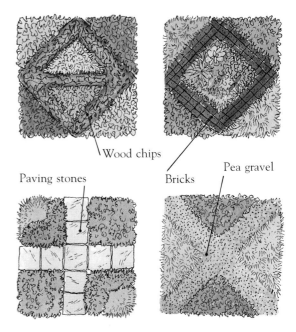

Wood chips

Paving stones

Pea gravel

Bricks

▲ **Use pathways** *as design elements. Choose paving that complements your herbs' colors and textures.*

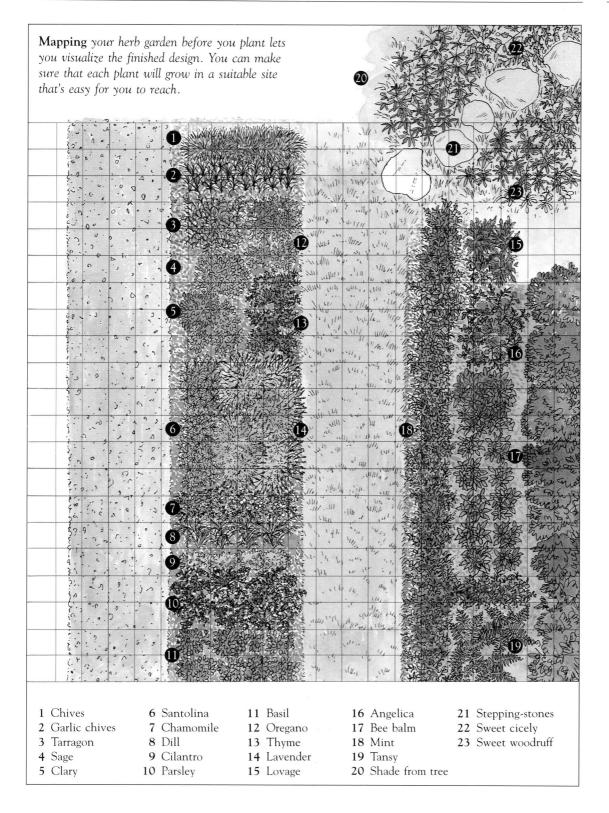

Mapping *your herb garden before you plant lets you visualize the finished design. You can make sure that each plant will grow in a suitable site that's easy for you to reach.*

1 Chives	6 Santolina	11 Basil	16 Angelica	21 Stepping-stones
2 Garlic chives	7 Chamomile	12 Oregano	17 Bee balm	22 Sweet cicely
3 Tarragon	8 Dill	13 Thyme	18 Mint	23 Sweet woodruff
4 Sage	9 Cilantro	14 Lavender	19 Tansy	
5 Clary	10 Parsley	15 Lovage	20 Shade from tree	

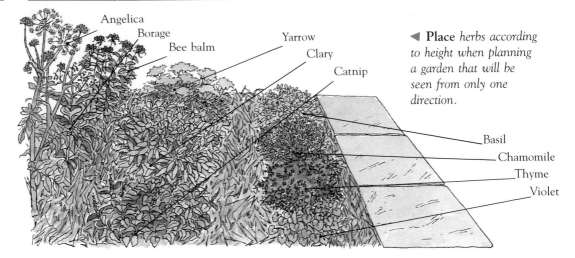

Angelica
Borage
Bee balm
Yarrow
Clary
Catnip

◀ **Place** *herbs according to height when planning a garden that will be seen from only one direction.*

Basil
Chamomile
Thyme
Violet

three wormwoods on the wide end and one on the narrow side can pull it together.

Edgings: Edgings also unify gardens. If your herb garden is small, you may want to edge the entire area with a low-growing, adaptable plant such as thyme. If this is impractical, you can also use bricks, rocks, slate, wood, or other materials for the edging. In an herb garden with brick pathways, for example, a series of upright, angled bricks, buried to their midpoints, will define and unify the space.

Enclosures: Almost everyone loves enclosed gardens, but few of us are lucky enough to have a couple of old stone walls hanging around the property. Fortunately, it's easy to create a sense of enclosure with hedges or fences. If you want to make the garden enclosure do double duty, set up trellises as the garden "walls" and plant small fruits along them. Raspberries, blackberries, and grapes are good choices for these trellises.

Illusion of depth and size: Illusion is as easy to create in a garden as it is on the canvas. The wise use of color makes this possible. If you want to make your small garden space appear larger than it is, use a painter's trick. Place the plants with cool colors – blues, blue-greens, purples, and dark greens – toward the back of the garden. Put those with warm colors – bright yellows, oranges, pinks, reds, and yellow-greens – at the front. Cool colors tend to recede in our vision while warm ones

come forward. Size also plays a part in creating the sense of distance. Placing large-leaved plants at the rear of the garden and small, delicate-leaved plants in the front will contribute to the look of depth. (See "Color" on page 26 for more on using color.)

DESIGNING FOR CONVENIENCE

A few basic design guidelines will make it easy to care for your garden. Consider mulch, plant spacing, and pathways as you plan your garden.

Mulch matters: Mulches, discussed on page 43, can minimize and even eliminate weeding chores. Choose your mulch when you're planning the design. Because of visual considerations, your choice of mulching material influences the distance you leave between plants. Plants surrounded by a shallow, fine-textured mulch can be spaced more closely than plants with a deep, coarse-textured mulch. For example, plants mulched with landscape cloth covered with a thin layer of wood chips can grow as closely as they would without mulch. But straw mulches must be piled 6 to 8 inches deep; plants with this mulch will look better if they are spaced farther apart than usual – about 1½ times their spread.

Plant spacing: Herbs grow to mature size quickly, so be sure to give them enough elbowroom right from the start. If you space plants appropriately, they'll have enough space to grow for at least

▶ **Control** *invasive herbs like mint by planting them in pots sunken into the garden soil.*

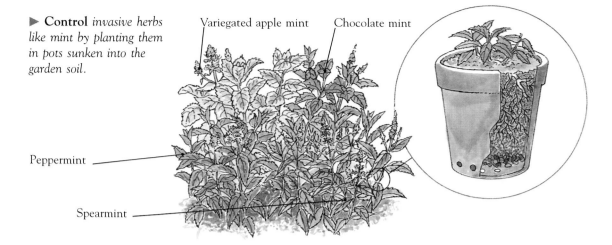

Variegated apple mint   Chocolate mint

Peppermint

Spearmint

three years before they need dividing. Properly spaced plants will also help to shade out weeds growing between them. Look in the Directory, beginning on page 98, to learn how wide each of your herb plants will spread, and use that figure while you're planning the design.

The garden path: Design your pathways so you can reach every plant in the garden. If you are using the shape of paths to help define the form of the garden, you can heighten this effect by using a different mulch material or even paving stones on them. Almost everyone is most comfortable working from pathways that measure at least 2 feet wide. If your garden will include creeping plants along the path edges, allow a width of 2½ feet.

If you've designed a very wide bed and don't want to break it up with pathways, use large stones set into the soil at intervals close enough so that you can comfortably reach every spot of bare ground from one or another of them. Be sure you can reach every stone from either a pathway or another stone, as well. Keep in mind that stones can be weed catchers. If your garden is in newly turned soil where weedy grasses recently grew, they'll tend to reappear in the compacted soil at the edges of the stones. Wind-borne weed seeds will tend to lodge in niches close to the stones, too. Catch these interlopers while they're young for easy removal. On the other hand, seeds from your invited herbs will most likely sprout by the stones, too, softening the edges as they grow.

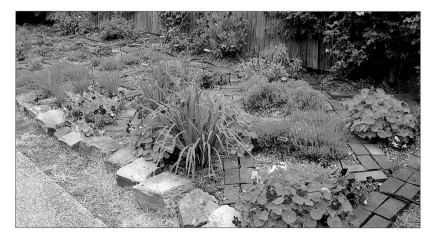

◀ **Bricks** *laid on the soil surface in this garden give easy access to the plants and allow some design flexibility as the plants mature.*

Formal Designs

If you love formal gardens, there's no better way to start one than with herbs. Despite appearances, a well-designed formal garden is much easier to care for than a natural-looking one, primarily because each plant group has such a well-defined area in which to grow.

As with any other kind of garden, the secret to making a manageable formal garden is scale. Start with a size that you can easily maintain. You can always expand later as you find new herbs you want to grow.

Knot gardens are one of the most traditional formal designs. In the seventeenth century, when every estate owner hired gardeners, these designs were at the pinnacle of their popularity. Hedges of slow-growing, compact shrubs with small leaves were planted in an interwoven pattern. Keeping them neat required meticulous pruning, both in the late winter and during the summer.

Knot gardens may seem impractical today, when none of us have an army of gardeners at the ready. But if you choose the plants carefully, you can use a knot design as the foundation plan for a contemporary garden. Many herbs grow so compactly, and keep themselves so tidy, that they are ideal for the interwoven hedges of a knot garden. They require little or no pruning to keep them in shape.

Among the plants in this category are 'Silver Mound' artemisia, the dwarf santolina 'Nana', 'Hidcote' and 'Munstead' lavender, and dwarf cultivars of rue. If you garden in the southern half

▶ **Knot designs,** *both opened and closed, are planted in the herb gardens at England's Hatfield House, where Queen Elizabeth I once lived.*

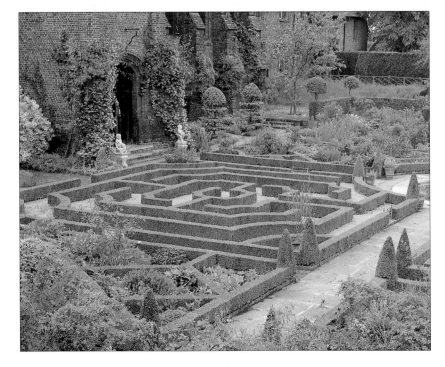

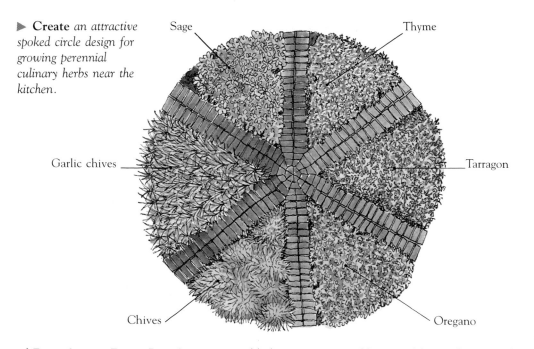

▶ **Create** *an attractive spoked circle design for growing perennial culinary herbs near the kitchen.*

Sage   Thyme

Garlic chives   Tarragon

Chives   Oregano

of Zone 6 or in Zones 7 or 8, you can add the relatively hardy 'Arp' rosemary to this list. Each of these plants may need a little pruning in early spring and midsummer, but they won't require the extensive maintenance of knot gardens of old.

These plants will make an interesting "open" knot garden, with the spaces between the hedges left unplanted so that the knot is the garden. If your taste runs to a more complicated design, you can plant a "closed" knot garden by interplanting other herbs between the hedges. Try a collection of small cultivars of thyme, such as silver thyme, golden lemon thyme, French thyme, woolly thyme, and German thyme. All retain a small, compact habit and their colors will complement the textures and colors of the hedges.

You can also use plants with a more relaxed or unruly habit, such as sage and hyssop, in easy-to-maintain formal designs. Without the formality of hedges and knots, you'll need to use man-made materials to provide the necessary structure for a garden with these more casual plants. Use weathered boards, bricks, or tiles to build a geometric pattern and fill it in with a variety of plants. But remember that these materials will be

a very visible part of the garden, so make sure you use appealing colors and designs.

Most formal gardens are composed of perennials because they take less maintenance in the long run, and the garden design can stay the same from year to year. But annual herbs, which you'll probably want to grow anyway, make an equally beautiful formal design. For example, the dwarf 'Spicy Globe' basil forms such a perfect sphere that it makes an ideal edging or dividing "hedge" for a formal planting. Sweet marjoram, summer savory, parsley, and other basils are also good herbs for formal gardens just as long as they are harvested often enough to keep them tidy-looking.

If you use annual plants, it's best to change the location of the annuals or the garden every year so pests and diseases don't have an opportunity to build populations. As you rotate it around your property, you may discover a place where it looks so good that it will inspire you to install a formal perennial garden there. And meanwhile you can take the opportunity to experiment with designs and colors using new annuals every year.

Kitchen Gardens

Kitchen gardens were once large enough to hold all the fruits, vegetables, and herbs, both medicinal and culinary, that a house-hold used through the year. Traditionally, they were sited at the rear of the house and enclosed by walls, because our ancestors thought them too utilitarian to be on public display.

BEAUTY AND CONVENIENCE

Thomas Jefferson, who was as innovative a gardener as he was a statesman, was the first American of note to install his kitchen garden where every casual visitor could easily see it. Fortunately for contemporary gardeners, his approach has prevailed. Today kitchen gardens are designed as much for their ornamental value as their usefulness.

Siting is still number one when it comes to herbs for the kitchen garden. You'll want to grow your kitchen herbs close to the house to make spur-of-the-moment picking easy.

Ideally, you'll be able to grow all the herbs that like hot, dry soil in a bed to the south side of your doorway, while you grow the rest in cool, moist soil under the filtered shade of a nearby tree or where the house gives them afternoon shade. In reality, you'll probably be growing some kitchen herbs farther than a few steps from your stoop. An alternative is to grow the culinary herbs you use most frequently in containers. (See "Growing Herbs Indoors" on page 50 for tips on container-grown herbs.) Even if you are surrounded by pavement, you can set the containers where light conditions are most suitable for your plants and also where they're convenient to the kitchen.

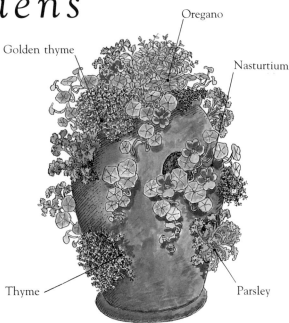

Golden thyme   Oregano   Nasturtium

Thyme   Parsley

▲ **Strawberry jars** *make wonderful containers for culinary herbs. Use a collection of herbs that require similar light and moisture levels.*

HOW MUCH IS ENOUGH?

Newcomers to herb gardening are often surprised at the large quantities that a single herb plant can produce. Just one mature tarragon plant, for example, can satisfy a family's culinary needs all through the year, even giving enough for a few quarts of tarragon vinegar. One rosemary plant is all you need for cooking (but if you use the leaves in potpourris, you might want several plants).

If you preserve herbs by freezing or drying, you'll want to account for this in your plan. For example, a year's worth of pesto in the freezer might require as many as a dozen basil plants and, depending on your recipe, as many as six parsley plants. Winter supplies of herbal teas also require larger numbers of plants. As you gain experience with the individual herbs, you'll learn how much of each to grow. But as a beginning, the chart opposite can serve as a guide.

HOW MUCH SHOULD YOU PLANT?

Herb	For Cooking	For Tea or Preserving	Herb	For Cooking	For Tea or Preserving
Angelica	1 plant	1 plant	Lavender	2 plants	6–12 plants
Anise (for seeds)	6 plants		Lemon balm	4 plants	6–12 plants
Anise hyssop	2–3 plants	8–12 plants	Lemongrass	2 clumps	
Basil	4–6 plants*	8–12 plants	Lemon verbena	3–4 plants	10–12 plants
Bee balm		6 plants	Lovage	1 plant	1 plant
Betony	1–2 plants	6–12 plants	Marjoram	2–4 plants	6–10 plants
Borage	1 plant	2–4 plants	Mints	1–2 plants	8–12 plants
Calendula	6 plants	12 plants	Nasturtium	6–8 plants	
Caraway	6 plants	12 plants	Oregano	2–4 plants	6–12 plants
Catnip		12 plants	Parsley	6 plants	12–18 plants
Chamomile		40–60 plants	Rosemary	1 plant	2–3 plants
Chervil	6 plants*	12 plants	Saffron crocus		50 plants
Chives	4 clumps	6 clumps	Sage	1–2 plants	4–6 plants
Cilantro	12 plants*	20–40 plants	Savory, summer	2–4 plants	6–8 plants
Clary	1 plant	6 plants	Savory, winter	2–4 plants	6–8 plants
Dill	10 plants*	20–40 plants	Tarragon	1 plant	2–3 plants
Fennel	1–2 plants	4–5 plants	Thyme	6 plants	12–18 plants
Hyssop	2 plants	12–36 plants			

*Total number, divided between successive plantings

▶ **Plant** *a succession of quickly maturing herbs such as dill to ensure a steady supply.*

Flowering plants being harvested

Seedlings to be transplanted into the same area

Herbs for Fragrance

*What could be more wonderful
than sweet-smelling herbs?
It's such a pleasure to
walk through a garden
where shifting breezes
carry fresh fragrances, or to
pick a bouquet of scented herbs,
or to create potpourris and aromatic
winter displays. It's difficult to imagine
an herb garden without these treasures.*

Think about ways to incorporate fragrant plants when planning your herb garden. Some people group together all those that love cool, moist soil and have another garden for those that like sunny, drier conditions. Others interplant them with the culinary herbs and in the vegetable garden. Either way, be sure to save some room for fragrant herbs.

Lavender is one of the most enjoyable and easiest plants to grow. Gardeners in Zone 6 and warmer can grow a whole garden of nothing but lavenders, each of them different from the rest. Good herb supply houses carry more than a dozen different types. Some of these plants have a more camphorlike odor than the familiar sweet-smelling varieties. Others have pink or violet flowers, fernlike or woolly leaves, or even bright green foliage. In Zones 3, 4, and 5, 'Hidcote', 'Munstead', and 'Lavender Lady' are reliably winter-hardy if insulated with deep mulch or snow. A patch of these three cultivars makes a beautiful display that's well worth the extra attention of tucking them in for the winter.

Both scented geraniums and mints also come in more cultivars than you probably imagine. You can treat yourself to a wonderful sampler garden of just scented geraniums, or of just mints. Though the plants have distinctly different appearances, they complement each other beautifully.

Scented geraniums grow rapidly from young plants and quickly reach a good size in the garden. They're tender perennials, extremely sensitive to cold and frost. Many gardeners in colder climates plant them in the garden as annuals, enjoying them during the spring, summer, and early fall. Some gardeners prune back and pot up the plants when frost threatens, wintering them indoors on a sunny windowsill. Others simply grow their scented geraniums in pots year-round. The variety of foliage textures and soft colors combine beautifully with terracotta. It's fun to set a collection of potted plants on a porch or balcony where you can brush against their deliciously fragrant leaves.

Think long and hard before you select a location for mints in the garden. They have earned their aggressive reputation. Even planted with other mints, they can be wildly invasive. If you are willing to let mints compete among themselves, give them a bed far away from other

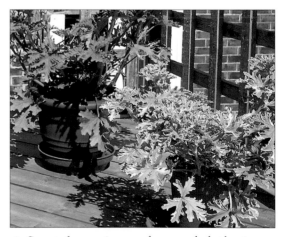

▲ **Scented geraniums** *enhance a deck planting where their fragrant leaves are within easy reach.*

FRAGRANT HERBS		
Herb	*Part Used*	*Use*
Bee balm	Leaves and flowers	Bouquets, potpourris
Clary	Leaves	Bouquets, potpourris
Geraniums, scented	Leaves and flowers	Potpourris, sachets
Lavender	Leaves and flowers	Bouquets, potpourris, sachets, dried arrangements
Lemon balm	Leaves	Bouquets, potpourris
Lemongrass	Leaves	Potpourris, sachets
Lemon verbena	Leaves	Potpourris, sachets
Marjoram, sweet	Leaves	Potpourris, sachets
Mints	Leaves	Potpourris, sachets
Rosemary	Leaves	Potpourris, sachets
Santolina	Leaves and flowers	Bouquets, potpourris, dried arrangements
Southernwood	Leaves	Bouquets, sachets, dried arrangements
Sweet woodruff	Leaves	Potpourris, sachets
Wormwood	Leaves	Bouquets, sachets, dried arrangements

plants and install a sunken, foot-deep barrier of plastic or galvanized metal to help keep them confined. (Mulching around the edges of a mint bed will slow them down, but they'll soon scoot under it to pop up in the grass on the other side.) An alternative is to plant your mints in sunken buckets, as illustrated on page 19.

Lemon verbena, lemongrass, and rosemary are also good potted plants for gardeners in cold-winter areas. Lemon verbena has graceful trailing and branching stems and makes a lovely hanging basket plant. Lemongrass grows in an upright clump of dense, grassy leaves that are a delight to sniff. Rosemary cultivars offer a variety of beautiful forms. You can train trailing types to form small topiaries, while bushy plants acquire a bonsai-like appearance as they age. Rosemary appreciates heat so much that you can set its pot on a sunny, concrete porch without a worry.

Southernwood is a wonderfully large, beautiful plant. When you brush against the foliage, it releases a clean, camphorlike odor. Some people, and all moths, are repelled by this scent, but others love it. Since the plant grows to 5 feet high and spreads at least 2 feet, you'll only need one. If you like the fragrance, plant it where you'll brush against it as you enter the garden.

Have some fun experimenting with the fragrant herbs. They'll add a wonderful dimension to your herb garden. Once you discover how easily you can use them to make scented oils, toiletries and potpourris, and other fragrant crafts, you'll want to keep adding to your collection.

▶ **Grow** *herbs with similar cultural needs together.*

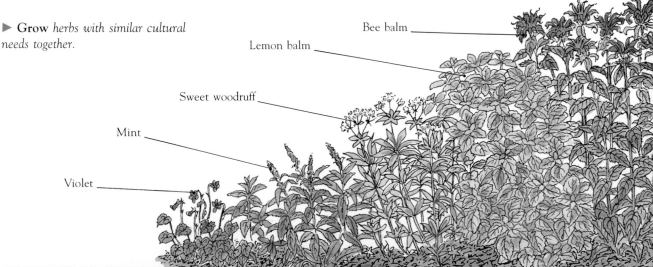

Bee balm

Lemon balm

Sweet woodruff

Mint

Violet

Color

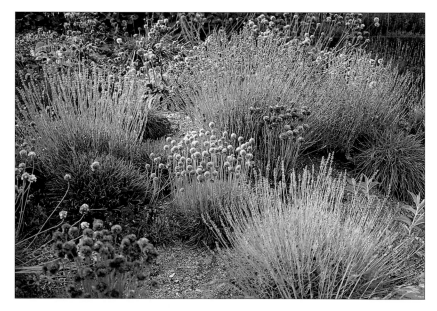

Before you grow herbs, you may think of them as being a generic sort of "green" color, but your first herb garden will change that idea. Color is as strong an element in herb gardens as it is in a perennial border. Herb foliage runs the gamut from deep blue-greens through silvers, grays, and yellow-greens. Added to this spectrum are the many herbs with colored or variegated leaves and the ones with brightly colored blooms.

W hen you are planning the herb garden, think about the colors of the herbs as well as their dimensions and environmental requirements. Though most herbs complement each other, you'll create a more pleasing garden if you divide patches of the strongly colored plants with clear green herbs such as standard sweet basil, betony, catnip, chervil, cilantro, lemon balm, parsley, pennyroyal, the savories, and valerian.

Clear greens are particularly important when you include variegated plants in the herb garden. Some of these, such as golden lemon thyme, golden-feather feverfew, and variegated rue, have leaves with complementary or similar coloration. While it might be tempting to group them together, the effect is so overwhelming that you barely notice the individual plants and the balance of the garden is thrown off. Instead, try to use patches of variegated herbs as focal points. They have so much visual punch that a "chain" of them, broken up by clear green herbs, can lead the eye from one side of the garden to the other.

Silver- and gray-leaved plants can also play a special role. Like white-flowered plants, they brighten any area where they grow. If you have a corner in partial shade, for example, the soft silvery foliage of wormwood will light up the area.

▶ **Blooming herbs** *can be as spectacular as any other ornamentals. Here, mauve-colored chive flowers complement the fragrant spikes of lavender.*

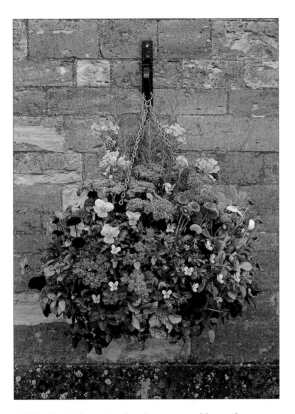

▲ **Herbs in hanging baskets** *can add a welcome – and portable – splash of color.*

FLOWER COLORS

Although many herbs have flowers that are barely noticeable, a few have vividly colored blooms. Sage and lavender flowers, for example, range from bright pinks to intensely deep purples. Calendula, with its orange and bright yellow blooms, will clash with some of the pink and purple shades. Use plants with clear green or blue-green foliage to separate its hot colors from other brightly colored neighbors.

Nasturtiums come in a range of mostly fiery colors. They can make a good companion to purple-flowered sages, but those hot nasturtium orange and orange-yellow colors aren't good with red-flowered pineapple sage or any of the bee balms. 'Cambridge Scarlet' bee balm is such a vivid red that it dominates other colors, even if

you put it toward the rear of an herb bed. Planting white-flowered feverfew at its base will make the color stronger; the blue-green of rue foliage will mute it somewhat.

Sometimes, in spite of all your planning, you'll find that you have a color scheme that clashes. If you discover that you've made a mistake, don't hesitate to dig up and move the offending plant early in the following spring.

HERBAL FOLIAGE COLORS

Blue-green:	Colored or variegated:
Chives	Basil, opal
Garlic chives	Basil, 'Purple Ruffles'
Hyssop	Comfrey, variegated
Rue	Fennel, bronze
Gray-green:	Feverfew, 'Golden-
Borage	Feather'
Catnip	Geraniums, scented
Clary	(many varieties)
Geranium, rose-	Lemon balm, golden
scented	Mint, chocolate
Lavender, French	Mint, ginger
Mint, apple	Mint, pineapple
Sage	Rue, variegated
Southernwood	Sage, golden
Thyme, 'Tiny-leaf'	Sage, purple
Silver-gray:	Sage, tricolor
Santolina	Thyme, golden
Thyme, woolly	lemon
Wormwood	Thyme, silver

Basil, sweet

Basil, opal

Chapter

2

GROWING AND CARING FOR YOUR HERBS

❧

THIS CHAPTER *answers the sorts of questions that can make all the difference between enjoying your herb gardening tasks or being frustrated by them. In it, you'll learn how to provide the very best growing conditions for the different herbs you choose to grow. You'll find easy and effective ways to transform a section of your yard from lawn to good garden soil. Know what to look for when you shop for herb plants for your garden, and learn how to start your own herbs from seed, indoors or out. Mulching tips will save you time when it comes to weeding, watering, and improving the soil. And putting a stop to the occasional pest or disease problem is safe and easy with handy charts that show you what to look for and what to do. When you're ready to share your herbs with friends, learn which herbs you can divide and how to save seeds for next year's crop. Finally, include some time for fall cleanup in your gardening schedule, and enjoy the benefits of a healthier garden in the coming spring.*

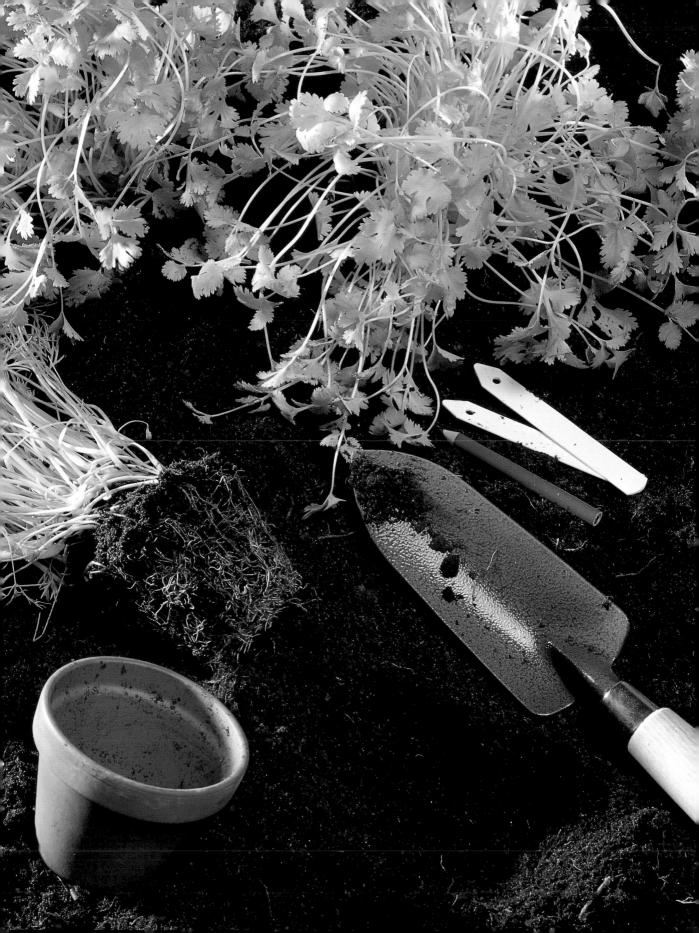

Breaking Ground

Good soil is truly the sturdy foundation upon which you'll build your healthy herb garden. But soil does much more than give your herbs physical support. It's also a storehouse of the nutrients, water, and air your plants need in order to thrive.

Good soil is alive with a bustling population of soil organisms that help turn decomposing plant matter into humus and help to protect your herbs against certain pests and diseases. Healthy, well-tended soil can make the difference between an herb garden that struggles along and one that flourishes with very little care from you.

Since few of us are lucky enough to start with a piece of land where the soil is already "good," our first step in making a beautiful herb garden is soil building. Establishing a new garden usually means either converting part of your lawn to a garden area or reworking an old garden area. In either case, start with the soil to create a healthy, productive, and attractive herb garden.

MAKING THE BED

Once you've decided on a style for your new garden (see chapter 1 for all your style options), you're ready to outline the bed and break ground. If you want your garden to have a formal look and straight sides, you can mark off its outline by measuring carefully, setting stakes at the corners, and then stretching string from post to post. To create a more free-flowing outline for your garden, use a flexible garden hose or a length of rope to form a pleasing shape.

If you are starting your new herb garden in an area that's now lawn grass, your next step will be to remove the grass. Stripping sod is easier than it sounds, and rolling up the strips is surprisingly fast work. You can strip sod by hand if your garden is small, or you can rent a sod-stripping machine for a large area. You can also smother the grass with deep mulch, and then plant your herbs into the mulched bed. This is a low-labor process, but it takes time – you'll have to wait until the following spring before you can plant.

IMPROVING YOUR SOIL

Unimproved soils vary a great deal from one place to the next. Some are sandy and dry, while others may be moist, compacted clay. But no matter what kind of soil you start with, increasing the amount of organic matter it contains will improve it dramatically. Some sources of organic matter you might add to your soil include leaves, grass clippings, straw, compost, and manure, to name just a few. Microorganisms, earthworms, and other soil animals feed on organic matter, breaking it down into nutrients your plants can use. As they work, these soil dwellers also improve the soil in other ways.

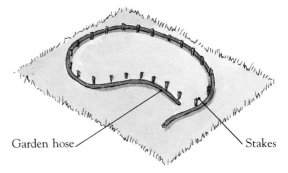

Garden hose   Stakes

▲ **A garden hose** *marks a graceful outline for a rounded garden. Use stakes to hold the hose in place, then sprinkle bonemeal around it to guide you when you dig.*

CREATE AN HERB GARDEN THE LOW-LABOR WAY

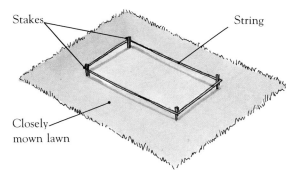

Stakes

String

Closely
mown lawn

▲ **Plan ahead** *to make a truly low-labor garden. Begin by mowing the lawn grass closely and then staking off the area.*

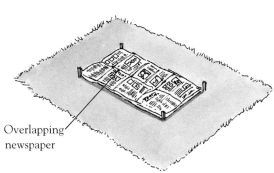

Overlapping
newspaper

▲ **Kill the grass** *by covering it with 1 to 2 inches of newspaper, overlapping the edges so the grass can't peek out.*

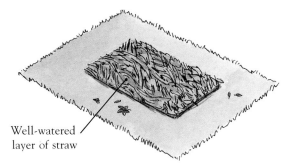

Well-watered
layer of straw

▲ **Water** *the newspaper to help hold it in place. Add 6 to 8 inches of straw, and water thoroughly.*

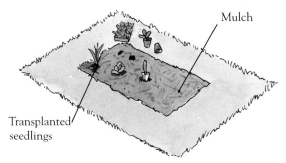

Mulch

Transplanted
seedlings

▲ **The following spring,** *transplant herbs into your new garden area. Mulch well to prevent weedy grasses from invading.*

Soils with high levels of organic matter become better soils because of:

Adequate aeration: Roots need oxygen as much as they need water. Soil animals and micro-organisms improve aeration by "gluing" small soil particles together into a crumb structure. The spaces between the soil crumbs hold air, which is vital to healthy roots. Boost the population of the soil critters by giving them organic matter to eat, and you naturally boost the amount of air in your

soil. You can see the proof of this with your own eyes: Just lift a handful of soil that's been improved with organic matter. Notice how light and fluffy it is, compared to unimproved soil.

Good moisture-holding capacity: Soils with a crumb structure hold more water than dense, compacted soils. After only a year of building humus levels by adding organic matter, you'll find that the soil retains moisture for greater periods of time. That means you can go longer between

▶ **Make** *a sod compost in layers, as shown. Let it sit for 7 to 10 days, then begin turning it as usual.*

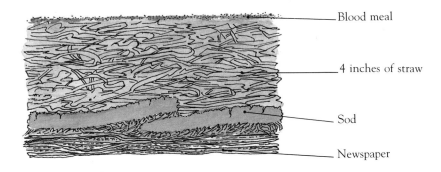

Blood meal

4 inches of straw

Sod

Newspaper

waterings when rainfall is scarce, because your plants' roots can draw more moisture out of the healthy, humus-rich soil.

Balanced and adequate nutrient content: Soils fertilized naturally, by the nutrients released from a variety of decomposed organic materials, tend to have a better nutritional balance than those fertilized with high concentrations of specific nutrients like nitrogen. Most organic materials release their nutrients slowly, allowing plants to take them up as they are needed, rather than in feast-or-famine doses. And most organic materials contain trace amounts of essential minerals and other substances that may be lacking in packaged fertilizers.

ADDING ORGANIC MATTER

Here are three great ways to add organic matter to your soil:

- Mulch with an organic material such as straw, rotted hay, or shredded leaves. (See "Mulching" on page 43 for more information.)
- Apply compost.
- Grow a cover crop and turn it under.

Growing a thick cover crop like buckwheat or clover, and then digging it into the soil as a "green manure," is one of the best ways to prepare the soil for an herb garden. This approach smothers weeds *and* adds a good amount of organic matter.

Cover crops work for both worn-out garden sites and areas of lawn that you're converting to garden. If you've already got a perennial herb garden, cover crops are hard to use – turning them in will disturb your herbs' roots. However, if you keep part of your garden for growing annual herbs, you can plant a winter cover crop every year to stop erosion, add organic matter, and suppress weeds.

FINE-TUNING FERTILITY AND pH

You'll find that herbs are an agreeable bunch of plants when it comes to soil fertility. Most grow just fine in average soil. A few herbs, such as nasturtiums, actually prefer soil that a vegetable gardener would consider poor and in need of improvement. If you're starting out with an average garden bed or a site where grass has grown well in the past, adding an inch or two of compost each year will probably supply enough nutrients to keep your herbs healthy. But if your intended herb garden is in a worn-out site or in a place where you know the soil is poor, start with a soil test to find out just what to add to get your herb garden up and running.

By analyzing both fertility and soil pH – the measure of its acidity or alkalinity, expressed as a number from 1 to 14 – before you plant, you'll be able to prepare the soil to the liking of your favorite herbs. And since you'll need to mix any fertilizers or other amendments thoroughly into the soil, the best time to adjust the pH balance and add nutrients is before you plant.

Take soil samples as directed by your testing lab (see "Resources" on page 155 for a list of soil-

WEED CONTROL

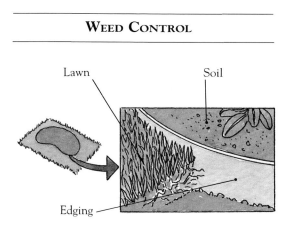

Lawn — Soil — Edging

▲ **Edge** *the garden to keep grass from invading.*

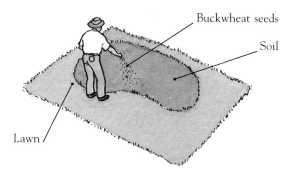

Buckwheat seeds — Soil — Lawn

▲ **Sow buckwheat** *seeds so they fall an inch or two apart.*

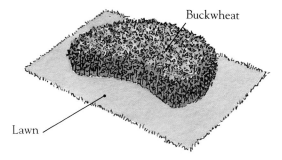

Buckwheat — Lawn

▲ **Buckwheat** *smothers weed seeds in the soil and restricts grass shoots by reducing the amount of light available. After the buckwheat sow winter rye. When it decomposes it kills many weed seedlings.*

testing laboratories) and have them analyzed for pH and the major and minor nutrients. For an herb garden, you'll want the pH to be between 6.3 and 7.1 – slightly acid to just above neutral (7.0 is neutral). If your soil's pH falls above or below this range, follow the lab's directions for adjusting it accordingly.

You may find that the soil in your new garden site is low in nutrients. In a new housing development, the topsoil may have been removed during construction. If you have stripped away the sod on top of your garden, you have also carried away some of the topsoil layer.

HOW MUCH FERTILIZER?

Your soil test will tell you the levels of major and minor nutrients in your garden bed. Before you fertilize, check your soil analysis against "Herbs at a Glance" on pages 9–12. Here you'll find which herbs prefer fertile soil and which prefer soil of low fertility. Most herbs grow well in soils with average fertility. You can safely assume that's the case where it's not specifically mentioned. If the analysis indicates that your soil falls in this average or moderate range, spread a $\frac{1}{2}$-inch layer of compost over the garden and mix it into the top 4 inches of soil. If the analysis measures soil nutrients as being low, apply 1 to 2 inches of compost to the area, mixing it into the soil to a depth of about 6 inches.

If the soil measures low in phosphates and potassium, apply rock powders along with the compost. Rock phosphate, applied at the rate of 30 to 50 pounds per 1,000 square feet, will supply phosphorus for four or five years. Potassium supplies are assured for the same length of time when you apply 50 to 100 pounds of greensand per 1,000 square feet.

Adding these three amendments – compost, rock phosphate, and greensand – at the start, and continuing with regular applications, will give your herb garden a good beginning and keep it healthy.

Transplants and Seeds

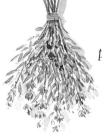

Planting is one of the most exciting parts of herb gardening. After all the planning and site preparation you've done, it's a wonderful feeling when you form the first furrow or transplant the first seedling.

Some herbs do best when their seeds are given an early start indoors. Other herbs are best grown from young plants that have been propagated vegetatively – by cuttings or divisions. And many grow easily from seed sown directly into your garden. Catalogs from reputable nurseries will often tell you which is which, and you can also consult the charts on pages 35 and 38. It's likely that you'll be transplanting some purchased plants, transplanting some seedlings you grew yourself, and seeding some herbs directly in the soil, all in the same garden.

STARTING SEEDS INDOORS

It's practical and fun to start many of your homegrown seedlings indoors. Thyme, oregano, and some other herbs are so tiny as seedlings that it's easy to lose track of them if you sow them outdoors. By starting them inside, you can grow them to manageable size before planting out. Other herbs, including betony, parsley, and rue, are very slow growing. You'll want to give them a head start indoors so they have time to grow to a good size in your garden.

Starting seeds indoors gives you a jump on the season, a useful trick with annual herbs. You'll want to sow your main crop of basil and other annuals directly in the garden. But by starting your first planting inside, you can harvest earlier

HERBS TO BUY AS PLANTS

Sometimes it's best to buy herbs as plants instead of growing them from seed yourself. Some herbs don't produce viable seeds. Other herbs can be grown from seed, but because you only need a few of them and they take so long to grow, it's more economical to buy a few small plants. Many cultivars don't come true from seed, although you may be able to grow the species type of the same herb from seed.

Golden sage, for instance, should be grown from a cutting or a young plant, but culinary sage will come true from seed. Similarly, all seed-grown mints share a typical minty flavor and make a good-tasting tea, but if you want a particular cultivar, such as orange mint, you'll have to buy a plant to be sure of getting the right flavor.

For the best results in your herb garden, start with plants of the following herbs:
Aloe
Comfrey, 'Bocking' cultivars
Geraniums, scented, many cultivars
Lavender, many cultivars
Lemon verbena
Mint, many types and many cultivars
Rosemary
Sage, many cultivars
Santolina, many cultivars
Southernwood
Tarragon
Thyme, many cultivars
Wormwood, many cultivars

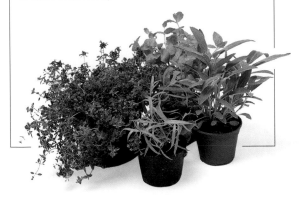

HERBS TO START FROM SEED INDOORS

These herbs are usually grown from seed started indoors and transplanted to the garden. Use this chart to learn when to sow, how to start them, and when it's safe to transplant them outdoors.

Herb	Starting Date	Germination or Starting Requirements	Transplant Outdoors
Angelica	July-August	Seeds are viable only when fresh, require light for germination, start in moist medium at 60°F	See Directory, page 101
Anise	March-April	Start in peat pots at 70°F	Frost-free date
Anise hyssop	March-April	Start in peat pots at 70°F	Frost-free date
Basil	April-May	Start in moist medium at 80°F	1 week after frost-free date
Bee balm	March-April	Start in moist medium at 75°F	1 week before frost-free date
Betony	March-April	Start in moist medium at 75°F	Frost-free date
Borage	March-April	Start in peat pots at 75°F	Frost-free date
Calendula	March-April	Start in moist medium at 70°–75°F	2 weeks before frost-free date
Chives	March-April	Start in moist medium at 70°F, seeds require darkness	2 weeks before frost-free date
Clary	March-April	Freeze 3-5 days before sowing, seeds require darkness, start in moist medium at 60°–65°F	1 week before frost-free date
Feverfew	April	Start in moist medium at 75°–80°F	2 weeks after frost-free date
Lavender	March-April	Seeds require light for germination, start in moist medium at 70°F	Frost-free date
Lemongrass	March-April	Start in moist medium at 75°–85°F	See Directory, page 126
Marjoram, sweet	March-April	Start in moist medium at 70°–75°F	Frost-free date
Mints	March-April	Start in moist medium at 70°–75°F	1 week before frost-free date
Oregano	March-April	Start in moist medium at 70°F	1 week before frost-free date
Parsley	March-April	See Directory, page 134	1 week before frost-free date
Rue	March	Start in moist medium at 75°F	Frost-free date, wait until seedlings are 2"-3" tall
Sage	March-April	Freeze 3-5 days before sowing, seeds require darkness, start in moist medium at 60°–65°F	1 week before frost-free date
Santolina	March-April	Start in moist medium at 75°F	Frost-free date
Sweet cicely		See Directory, page 144	
Tansy	March-April	Start in moist medium at 75°–80°F	Frost-free date
Thyme	March-April	Start in moist medium at 70°F	1 week before frost-free date
Valerian	March-April	Start in moist medium at 75°F	Frost-free date
Wormwood	March-April	Start in moist medium at 70°F	1 week before frost-free date

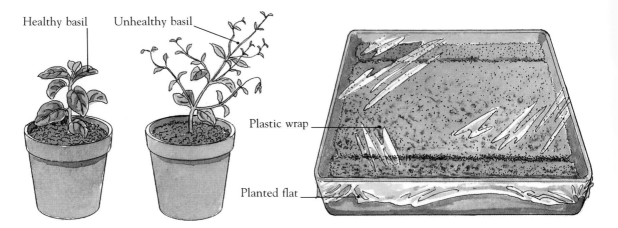

Healthy basil   Unhealthy basil

Plastic wrap

Planted flat

▲ **Choose** *"thrifty" seedlings – young plants with room to grow in their pots, short spaces between their branches, and healthy green color.*

▲ **Cover** *planted flats with plastic wrap to keep soil moisture levels high while seeds are sprouting. Remove the plastic as soon as plants germinate.*

in the season. If you want extra-early harvests of anise, chervil, cilantro, and dill, sow some seeds indoors a few weeks before your last spring frost date in pots made of peat, paper, or other plantable material.

Indoor seed starting is much easier than you might think. Success is almost always guaranteed if you:

● Pay attention to the germination requirements, including soil temperature, listed in "Herbs to Start from Seed Indoors" on page 35 and in the Directory entries, beginning on page 98.

● Keep the starting soil mix consistently moist.

● Set flats or pots where they get good air circulation and bright light once seedlings begin to appear.

Patience doesn't hurt either. Unlike most vegetables grown from seeds, some herbs may take a few weeks to germinate. Whenever you are starting a perennial you've never grown before, give the seeds at least three weeks to a month to sprout. During that time, keep the seed-starting medium moist and keep the container in the correct environment. If there's still no sign of life, check the germination requirements again. Some perennial herb seeds need very special treatment to convince them to start growing.

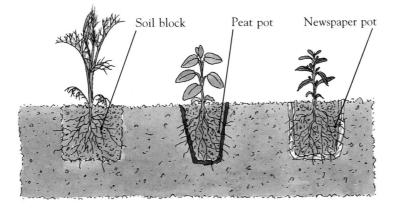

Soil block   Peat pot   Newspaper pot

◀ **Plant** *these pots and your transplants will adjust more easily to the outside garden.*

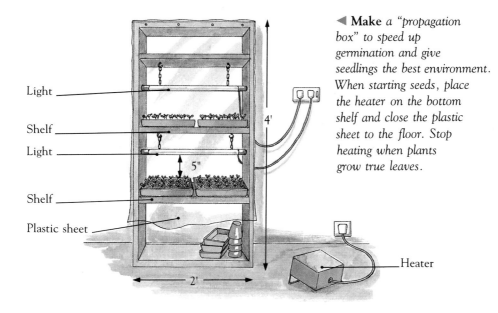

◀ **Make** *a "propagation box" to speed up germination and give seedlings the best environment. When starting seeds, place the heater on the bottom shelf and close the plastic sheet to the floor. Stop heating when plants grow true leaves.*

Light

Shelf

Light

Shelf

Plastic sheet

4'

5"

2'

Heater

Grow your seedlings at temperatures slightly cooler than those at which they were germinated. Indoor temperatures are usually warm enough but the air is often too dry. To increase humidity, mist the air around your seedlings every morning and, if possible, again in the early afternoon.

TRANSPLANTING INTO THE GARDEN

When you move your young herbs into the garden depends on the cold-hardiness of the plants. Check "Herbs to Start from Seed Indoors" on page 35 to learn when it's safe to transplant specific herbs. Keep in mind that you'll want to allow several days for "hardening off" your tender seedlings, a process of gradually exposing them to the conditions of the garden. The hardening-off illustrations below offer ideas and suggestions to help you introduce your seedlings to the outdoors.

Choose a cloudy day for transplanting, or wait until after 3 P.M., when the sun isn't as strong as earlier in the day. Before transplanting, soak each seedling's root ball in a mixture of 1 part seaweed and 1 part fish emulsion, each diluted according to label directions. After you plant your herbs, firm the soil well around each one to bring the roots into contact with the surrounding soil.

If you've purchased herb plants from a nursery or greenhouse, you can plant them in your garden

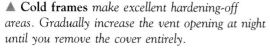

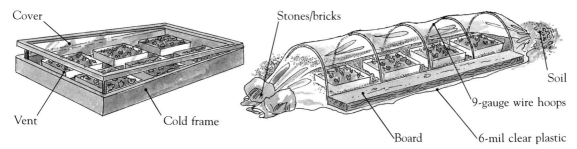

Cover

Vent

Cold frame

Stones/bricks

Soil

9-gauge wire hoops

Board

6-mil clear plastic

▲ **Cold frames** *make excellent hardening-off areas. Gradually increase the vent opening at night until you remove the cover entirely.*

▲**Plastic tunnels** *are inexpensive and practical. Harden plants by opening first one end, then the other. Finally, remove the plastic entirely.*

much as you would your own seedling transplants. The plants you buy will need hardening off too – how much they need depends on where they were growing when you bought them. Gradually move greenhouse-grown herbs outside, giving them time to adjust to cooler temperatures, wind, and increased light levels. Field-grown herbs, or those that have been held for a few weeks in an outdoor sales area, will be better prepared for planting directly into your garden. Keep your new purchases well watered until you're able to move them into the garden, and give them a preplanting soak in liquid seaweed and fish emulsion, as described on page 37.

SOWING DIRECTLY IN THE GARDEN

You can sow many herbs, even the perennial ones, directly into your garden soil. A little extra care in the beginning makes things easier in the long run.

Even if you've stripped away the sod or planted a cover crop one year in advance, weed seeds still lurk in the soil, just waiting for their chance to germinate. Deprive them of this opportunity by using the farmers' trick of making a "stale seedbed." Prepare the soil as usual by tilling and raking it. But don't plant right away. Instead, wait a week. During that time, weed seeds close to the surface will germinate. Kill them by drawing a

HERBS TO SOW WHERE THEY'LL GROW

There are many herbs that you can start from seed sown directly in the garden. Use this chart to learn when to start them and when to expect your first harvest.

Herb	First Planting	Second Planting	First Harvest
Angelica	July to August		Following summer
Anise	After frost-free date when soil is 70°F		Mid- to late summer
Anise hyssop	1 week before frost-free date		Midsummer to early fall
Basil	After frost-free date when soil is 70°F	Early to late July	2 months from sowing
Betony	1-2 weeks before frost-free date		Midsummer
Borage	After frost-free date		Late summer
Calendula	See Directory, page 109		3 months from sowing
Caraway	When soil can be worked		Late summer
Catnip	1-2 weeks before frost-free date		Late summer
Chamomile	When soil is 55°-60°F		Midsummer
Chervil	1-2 weeks before frost-free date	Mid- to late July	1½ months from sowing
Cilantro	After frost-free date	Every month until August	1½ months from sowing
Clary	1-2 weeks before frost-free date		Mid- to late summer
Dill	After frost-free date	Every month until August	1½ months from sowing
Fennel	1-2 weeks before frost-free date		Mid- to late summer

sharp hoe just under their tiny roots, no deeper than an inch below the soil surface. This technique eliminates the weeds close to the soil surface without bringing up weed seeds buried deeper in the soil. Wait until the following day to plant your seeds, and take care to disturb the soil as little as possible during planting.

To germinate, seeds need the right soil temperature (see "Herbs to Start from Seed Indoors" on page 35) and nearly constant moisture levels. When you are planting an herb that takes a long time to germinate, such as parsley, cover the planting rows with a couple of sheets of newspaper, weighted at the edges to keep them in place, and water thoroughly. The newspaper retains some moisture, allowing you to water only once a day during sunny periods. If the seeds require light for germination, cover them with floating row cover material instead of newspaper.

After your seeds have sprouted, thin them to an appropriate spacing. Some herbs, such as chives, dill, and thyme, grow well when sown thickly. Give larger, branching plants, such as anise hyssop, borage, and sage, enough space to grow to their full potential. Check the Directory, beginning on page 98, for the recommended garden spacing for each herb.

Herb	First Planting	Second Planting	First Harvest
Hyssop	1-2 weeks before frost-free date		Mid- to late summer
Lemon balm	1-2 weeks before frost-free date		Mid- to late summer
Lovage	Late summer or early fall		Following summer
Nasturtiums	After frost-free date		Midsummer
Pennyroyal	1-2 weeks before frost-free date		Mid- to late summer
Sage	1 week before frost-free date		Late summer
Santolina	1 week before frost-free date		Late summer
Savory	1 week before frost-free date		Mid- to late summer
Sweet cicely	See Directory, page 144		
Sweet woodruff	In early fall		Following summer
Valerian	1-2 weeks before frost-free date		See Directory, page 149
Vervain, European	1-2 weeks before frost-free date		Mid- to late summer
Wormwood	In early fall		Late August
Yarrow	1 week before frost-free date		July to August

Caring for Your Garden

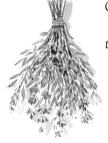

Care begins once your herbs are transplanted or have transformed themselves from small brown seeds into tiny green seedlings. If you've planned, prepared, and planted well, taking care of your herb garden won't require much time or effort. Until harvest begins, your only jobs are thinning, watering, weeding, and possibly mulching. In fact, caring for herbs is so easy, you'll probably want to expand your herb garden!

THINNING

As soon as your baby herbs have developed one or two sets of true leaves, it's time to thin them to the correct spacing distance. Check the entries in the Directory, beginning on page 98, to learn how much space each of your herbs needs.

Thinning gives the roots of each plant plenty of space to gather food and water. Overcrowded plants can't grow to their full potential because they're on a starvation diet. Jam-packed plants may also suffer from inadequate sunlight if they're being shaded by too-close neighbors.

Giving your herbs enough elbowroom also goes a long way toward ensuring plant health. All plants release moisture from their leaves. Unless a breeze is blowing, this moisture tends to remain close to the leaf, raising the relative humidity right around the plant. In shady or crowded conditions, these elevated humidity levels can lead to a variety of fungal and bacterial diseases. Thinning helps to avoid these problems.

There are two ways to thin your plants. The first way is to pull the extras from the soil, and the second is to cut them off just under the soil surface. Plants' roots spread more extensively than their leaves and stems, so it's important to pull seedlings before their roots are intertwined with those of their neighbors.

You might think that cutting off extraneous seedlings makes more sense. However, the open wound left after cutting is an open invitation to rot organisms. In most cases, these organisms remain on the dying plant. But in waterlogged soil or where many seedlings have been cut off, these organisms can build to populations that can put your other plants at peril. Why take chances? Thin by pulling instead.

SUCCESSION PLANTING

To harvest a steady supply of popular annual herbs, such as basil, cilantro, and dill, from your garden, you'll need to plant more than one crop of each. Because these herbs mature quickly, you'll need to spend some garden-tending time removing plants that are past their prime and replacing them with seedlings. See "Herbs to Sow Where They'll Grow" on page 38 to find out

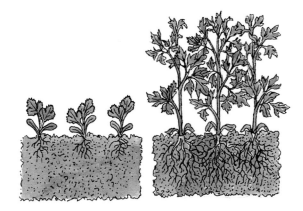

▲ **Thin** *young seedlings after they develop their first set of true leaves but before they grow so large that their once-individual root systems become a tangled mass of roots.*

► **Mulch** *can smother most of the weeds while also adding a decorative, finished look to your garden. Mulch perennials with bark; use straw or grass clippings for annual herbs.*

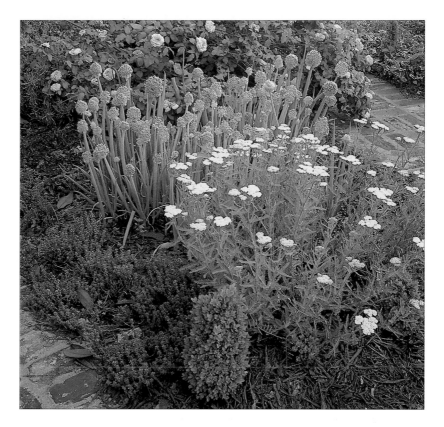

when to make second sowings of annual herbs to keep them producing throughout the summer.

WATERING

During the first season in a new garden, you'll learn how quickly the soil dries out and how frequently you need to water. The rate at which the soil dries depends on its type (sandy, silt, or clay), its humus content, the amount and intensity of the sunlight that hits it, and how windy the site is. Sandy, humus-poor soils, full sun exposure, and constant winds create fast-drying gardens. Humus-rich loams in partial shade and calm air retain soil moisture.

As you tend the plants in your herb garden, you'll begin developing a "water sense" about the soil. It's a good idea to develop the habit of checking once a day whenever seeds are germinating and at least every other day after they are established. As the garden changes over the

season, watering requirements do too. That's because the seasonal needs of your herbs will vary – in summer, they drink a lot; in fall, as they're going dormant, their water needs diminish. How you garden can affect how much you water too. For example, mulching decreases water loss, so you won't have to water as often.

Don't ignore the advice to water deeply when you water. Plants growing in beds where only the surface of the soil is really watered don't develop the deep roots they need to anchor themselves in the soil. Such plants are also more susceptible to drought damage when you do forget to irrigate.

Drip irrigation systems and soaker hoses save time as well as water. Be sure to set the timer to water deeply every few days instead of just a little bit every day. Check the moisture levels before you turn off your irrigation system. The soil should be moist to at least 8 inches deep.

If you water with a hose or a watering can, try

to be just as thorough. Water deeply – to moisten the soil to 8 inches or more below the surface – every few days, rather than sprinkling the soil surface every day.

Timing is also important. Try to water early in the morning. That way, leaves can dry before nightfall, and moisture can soak into the soil rather than evaporate into the air during the heat of the day. Watering early also helps prevent fungal disease problems, because the leaves dry quickly rather than staying wet and encouraging the growth and spread of these diseases.

WEEDING

Weeding destroys the competition in your herb garden. It gives your plants plenty of room to grow and abundant food and water, and it cuts down on disease and insect problems. Weeding also has the added benefit of making the garden look more beautiful.

The key to staying ahead of the weeds is just that – staying ahead of them. Weed early and often during the first part of the season. Once your herb garden is prepared, planted, and weeded, avoid turning the soil unnecessarily. Every time you bring soil up from beneath the surface, you'll expose new weed seeds to light, allowing them to sprout and grow amid your herbs. So use your hoe sparingly and with care, and pull out individual weeds with as little digging as possible to help keep weeds in check.

You'll find that weeds tend to come up in batches. The first weeds of the spring are the winter annuals that germinated the fall before and were so small then that you hardly noticed them. Next come the cool-season weeds, and then, just about the time you think you're finished with the major weeding of the year, there's a flush of frost-sensitive heat-lovers.

Fortunately, you do finally come to the end of major weeding chores. By July, the supply of weed seeds close to the surface will be so diminished that the large leaves of your herbs will shade most of the stragglers out. And by August, weeding is

LANDSCAPE FABRIC

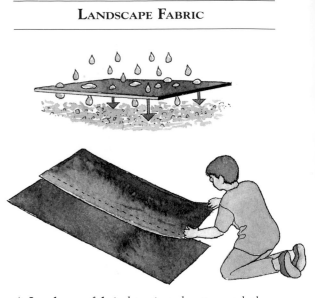

▲ **Landscape fabric** *lets air and water reach the soil while blocking weeds' growth. Overlap the fabric's edges in wide beds.*

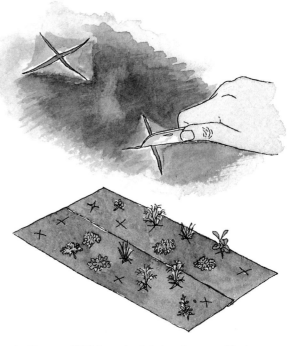

▲ **Cut an "X"** *into the fabric where you'll plant each seedling. Top the fabric with a layer of mulch to give your garden a finished look.*

only a memory for most gardeners. But don't ignore the tiny rosettes of winter annuals that begin appearing then. If you pull them this year, they won't be around next spring.

If you want to cut down on the time you spend weeding, there's a simple solution: mulch.

MULCHING

Mulches drastically cut weeding time by preventing weed seeds from getting the light they need to grow. The most effective mulches include landscape cloth, usually covered with a layer of wood chips; wood chips alone; shredded leaves; and straw. You can use a layer of newspaper under any of these mulches to block weed growth even more. Don't use grass clippings as a mulch around your perennial herbs. Grass clippings release a great deal of nitrogen as they decompose, so save them for annual herbs that will appreciate the additional nourishment.

Mulch the soil around plants that like cool growing conditions as soon as they are several inches taller than the intended mulch. Generally, that means your plants will be about 6 inches tall when you apply the first 2- to 3-inch mulch. For heat-loving plants, wait until the soil has warmed so you don't cool them down unnecessarily.

To avoid encouraging slugs and snails and other pests that love mulches, leave a 6- to 8-inch circle of bare soil around plant stems and leaf rosettes. You'll have to weed these bare spots by hand, but that's better than losing your plants to these pests.

The bottom layer of an organic mulch will gradually decompose, thanks to active populations of microorganisms turning the mulch into humus. This is great for the garden, but it does mean that you'll probably have to replenish your mulch during the growing season.

▼ **Mulching** *your tea garden makes it easier to care for and harvest from.*

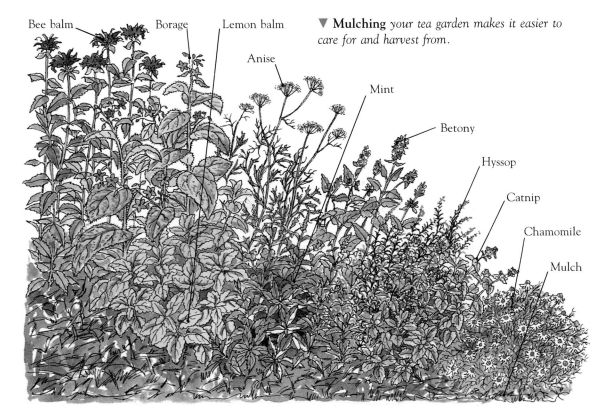

Bee balm   Borage   Lemon balm

Anise

Mint

Betony

Hyssop

Catnip

Chamomile

Mulch

Propagating Your Herbs

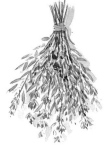

Multiplying your herbs by layering, division, and taking cuttings is a wonderfully easy way to increase your plants and expand your own garden for free or share your favorite plants with friends.

You'll find that layering, dividing, and rooting cuttings are all easier and more surefire ways for starting many herbs than planting seeds.

Spring is the best time to propagate most herbs, except in areas with very mild winters, where herbs can be propagated almost year-round. The level of light and the length of the day in spring, combined with warming temperatures, stimulate plant growth. Propagating in

PROPAGATION METHODS FOR HERBS			
Herb	Method	Timing	Comments
Aloe	Divide offshoots	Spring, early summer	See Directory, page 100
Bee balm	Divide plants	Early spring	Discard center growth
Catnip	Divide plants, cuttings	Early spring, or fall in Zones 6-9	
Chives	Divide plants	Spring, or fall in Zones 6-9	
Clary	Cuttings	Spring, early summer	
Comfrey	Divide roots	Early spring	
Geraniums, scented	Cuttings	Spring, fall	See Directory, page 121
Hyssop	Cuttings	Spring, early summer	
Lavender	Cuttings	Spring, early summer	
Lemon balm	Divide plants	Spring, early summer	
Lemongrass	Divide roots	Spring, early summer	See Directory, page 126
Lemon verbena	Cuttings	Spring, early summer	See Directory, page 127
Lovage	Divide plants	Spring, early summer	
Marjoram, sweet	Cuttings	Spring, early summer	
Mints	Divide plants, cuttings	Spring, early summer, or fall in Zones 6-9	
Oregano	Layer, cuttings	Spring, early summer	

spring also allows the new plant to become thoroughly established in the garden before winter begins.

Rosemary and tarragon are exceptions to this rule. Their cuttings are more likely to root if taken in the fall. Since it will be too cold to plant them outside after they have rooted, you can keep these herbs indoors until spring and then transplant them as usual.

See the illustrations for complete details on dividing and layering herbs and taking cuttings. "Propagation Methods for Herbs" below will tell you which methods will work best for multiplying your favorite herbs.

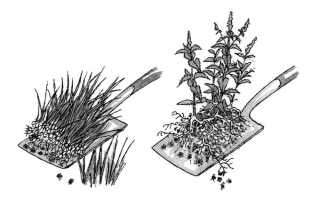

▲ **Dig** *entire root balls to divide herbs. Then pull roots like chives apart by hand, or cut fibrous root systems into two or three pieces.*

Herb	Method	Timing	Comments
Pennyroyal	Divide plants	Spring, early summer, or fall in Zones 6-9	
Rosemary	Cuttings	Fall	See Directory, page 136
Rue	Cuttings	Spring, early summer	
Saffron crocus	Separate new corms	Early summer	Divide every 3–4 years
Santolina	Cuttings	Spring, early summer	
Southernwood	Cuttings, divide plants	Spring, early summer	
Sweet cicely	Divide plants	Spring, early summer	
Sweet woodruff	Divide plants	Early spring	
Tansy	Divide plants	Spring, early summer, or fall	
Tarragon	Cuttings	Fall	See Directory, page 147
Thyme	Layer, cuttings, divide plants	Spring, early summer	
Valerian	Divide roots or crown	Spring	
Violet	Divide plants	Early spring	
Wormwood	Cuttings, divide plants	Spring, fall	
Yarrow	Divide plants	Spring	

TAKING CUTTINGS

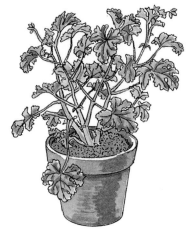 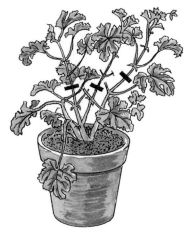 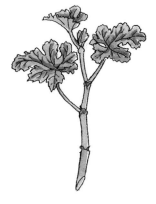

1 *Take cuttings of most herbs in the spring when they're growing rapidly.*

2 *Cut stems with at least five leaves. Cut on an angle, above an outward-facing leaf.*

3 *Remove the two bottom leaves and let the end of the stem dry for about 4 hours.*

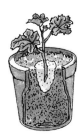 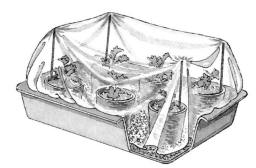 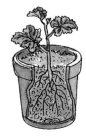

4 *Plant the stem in a channel of moistened vermiculite in a soil-filled pot.*

5 *Place the cuttings in a cool, low-light spot and drape with plastic for humidity.*

6 *New green leaves show that the roots have grown into the soil mix.*

LAYERING AND DIVISION

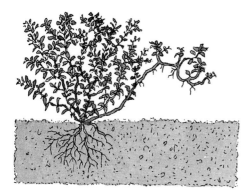

1 *Layer herbs with trailing stems. They'll root easily.*

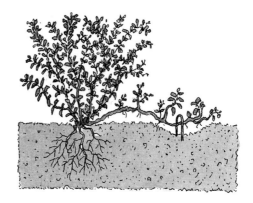

2 *Lay a long stem along the soil and pin it down.*

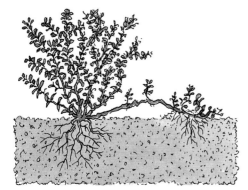

3 *New roots grow where the stem touches the soil.*

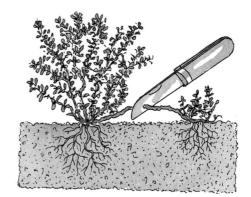

4 *Cut the stem after the new plant forms roots.*

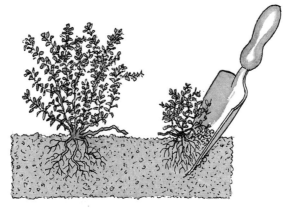

5 *Transplant young plants to their new locations.*

Preparing for Winter

Successful gardeners tend to think at least one season ahead, particularly when it comes to spring planting and winter preparation. Getting your herb garden ready for winter really begins in the late summer.

Perennial herbs withstand winter better if they have very little new growth as cold weather arrives. Since fertilizing them stimulates shoot and leaf production, it's wise to stop fertilizing, even with compost tea sprays, about one month before the first killing frost.

All but the last plantings of your annual herbs will begin to die back in late summer. Earlier in the year, you probably replaced annuals that were past their prime with new seedlings. But now, the final crop will soon be over, and it's time to think about protecting the soil over the winter.

Mulches and cover crops prevent your soil from eroding when winter rain runs off and snow melts. Although you might think of cover crops as an option only for large areas, such as entire growing beds, you can also use some cover crops in smaller spots.

For example, if small patches of annuals grew between perennials in your herb garden, a handful or two of oat seed is just what you need. When you've pulled out the annuals and composted them, scatter the oat seed on the soil, cover it lightly, and tamp it down. Within a week, bright green shoots will appear. The oats will die after the first heavy frost. Their dead leaves form a thick mulch that will hold the soil in place over the winter and retard early weed growth in the spring.

In all but the warmest climates, perennials should be mulched over the winter. Timing is important when applying this winter mulch. Mulches are insulating, keeping in both warmth and cold. The winter mulch will protect the plants' roots from severe cold and will keep the

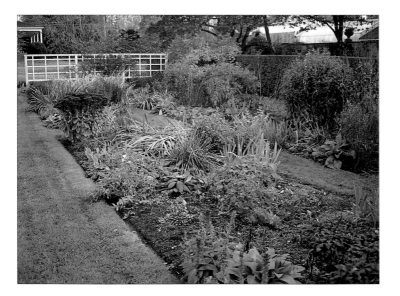

◀ **Cleaning up** *in fall makes the difference between a garden that thrives and one that just gets along. Rewards for cleanup come in spring.*

◀ **Clean** *your tools, then protect them from rust by plunging them into a pail of sand mixed with mineral oil.*

roots from heaving out of the ground during freezing-and-thawing cycles. Wait until the plant is securely dormant and about an inch of the ground is frozen before you mulch. When in doubt, wait until nighttime temperatures have been in the 20s for at least three days and daytime temperatures have been at freezing or below.

Straw, rotted hay, and shredded leaves are all good winter mulches. Pile about 8 inches of the mulch over the entire root area of the plant. If the garden is in a windy spot, weight down the mulch material with boards or pine boughs. Covering the mulch with a layer of burlap weighted down with stones or boards gives added protection for woody herbs such as southernwood or wormwood.

In very early spring, well before new growth has started, pull mulches back from the plants' crowns. It's best to leave the mulch material close at hand, though, because you may want to temporarily cover new growth if you get an unseasonable heavy frost or snowfall.

Wind can do as much damage during the winter as cold or freezing-and-thawing cycles. If your herb garden is in a windy place, you can protect plants from the worst of the winds by setting up wind barriers made from wooden stakes and burlap. In areas where the wind might come from any direction, set the stakes around the plants in a square or rectangular pattern, then staple burlap to the stakes. Where winds are only from one direction, a two-sided burlap shield with stakes set to form a corner around the plant will do. The burlap moderates the wind's drying effect on your plants.

Growing Herbs Indoors

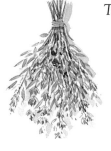

The thought of facing winter without a supply of fresh culinary herbs is enough to make many herb gardeners grow an indoor kitchen garden. Imagine fresh basil for midwinter tomato sauces or fresh sage for roast poultry

Most of us quickly discover that some of the easiest plants to grow in the outdoor summer garden are weak, spindly, and disappointing inside. In fact, very few herbs grow well just sitting in a little pot that's perched on the kitchen windowsill. But once you know a few tricks, your indoor herb garden success is almost guaranteed.

LET THERE BE LIGHT

Adequate light is all-important for herb plants inside. In most locations, sunlight isn't strong enough during the winter months to do more than just keep well-grown plants alive.

If you are growing a collection of herbs, buy a 4-foot-long fixture for fluorescent tubes. Cool white or daylight bulbs will work, but growth is stronger under full-spectrum plant tubes. Keep the tops of the plants no more than 5 inches from the tubes. To accommodate herbs of different heights, set their pots on individual wooden blocks or bricks to move them closer or farther from the light as necessary.

PLANNING YOUR INDOOR GARDEN

You can start your indoor herb garden from seed if you're growing annuals. To enjoy a taste of summer in your winter kitchen, start seed for

HERBS TO OVERWINTER INDOORS

A few of our favorite herbs just can't take the winters in most regions of the United States. To keep them from one year to the next, you'll have to overwinter them indoors, in a well-lit window or under a plant light. If you've planted them in pots, just bring in the pots for the cold months. If they are growing in the ground, you'll have to dig them and pot them up. Choose a pot that's at least 2 inches wider than the plant's root ball. You can take cuttings or make divisions of these plants too. In the right environment, cuttings will root and become established before spring.

In most regions, the following plants should spend the winter indoors:

Aloe	Lemon verbena
Geraniums, scented	Rosemary (hardy from
Lavender, French	Zone 8 south)
(*Lavandula dentata*)	Sage, pineapple
Lemongrass	Thyme, lemon

annual culinary herbs such as basil, chervil, cilantro, dill, and summer savory in mid- to late August. Plant about ten seeds around the edges of a 10- to 12-inch pot. After they germinate, thin to four or five plants. You can leave these pots outside for their first few weeks. To acclimate them to their winter quarters, move them into filtered shade at least a week before their big move indoors. Move tender annuals, especially basil, inside long before frost threatens.

When annual plants grow inside, even under artificial lights, they don't remain vigorous for as long as they do in the outside garden. For a

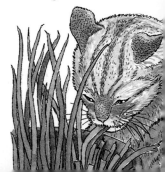

▶ **Satisfy** *herb-eating cats with a pot of grass for them to nibble.*

HERBS FOR A WINDOWSILL

These durable herbs are willing to spend the winter indoors growing on your windowsill without supplemental lighting. Although they'll grow more slowly during the winter, you'll still have a supply of fresh herbs to liven up your cooking. When spring arrives, transplant your windowsill herbs into the garden or move the pots outdoors.

Herb	Recommended Pot Size	Water Needs	Fertility Requirements	Light Requirements
Aloe	6–12 inches	Low	Medium	South window
Geraniums, scented	6–10 inches	Keep moist	High	South window
Lavender, French	6–12 inches	Keep moist	Medium	South window
Lemongrass	10–12 inches	Keep moist	Medium	South or east window
Lemon thyme	6–10 inches	Keep moist	Medium	South or east window
Lemon verbena	8–12 inches	Keep moist	High	South window
Mints	8–10 inches	Very moist	High	South or east window
Rosemary	8–12 inches	Slightly moist	Medium	South or east window
Sage, pineapple	8–12 inches	Keep moist	Medium	South or east window
Tarragon	8–12 inches	Keep moist	Medium	South or east window

constant supply, you'll want to plan on making successive plantings every four to six weeks, from October through February.

To have a supply of perennial herbs to snip from during the winter, you can pot up garden plants well before frost to bring them indoors. Pot up small divisions of perennials such as mint, oregano, tarragon, thyme, and winter savory when you divide them in the spring. Leave the pots outside all summer and through the early winter. These plants need the rest that a period of dormancy gives. In January, bring them into a slightly warmer area such as the basement or garage and leave them there for about a week. After that, bring them inside. Once growth has started, set them under the lights.

Chives also need to experience a winter rest. In the fall, plant divisions in pots at least 12 inches deep. Let them stay outside until January. Move them gradually into a heated area. Chives won't remain productive all winter, so pot up more than one bunch so you can bring the pots into the house one by one.

Parsley is particularly demanding when you bring it inside. The best way to handle this plant is to seed it directly into a pot in late June. You'll need a pot at least 12 inches deep by 12 inches wide. Keep the potted plant outside all summer, remembering to give it ample water and monthly feedings with compost tea solutions. Move the pot into filtered shade about a week before bringing it inside several weeks before frost threatens.

Pests and Diseases

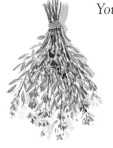

You won't find many pests in your herb garden. That's because the delightful fragrances that attract us so strongly to the herb garden have an opposite effect on many pests.

Insects and other pests are often repelled by plants with strong aromas, no matter how appealing they are to us. Because of this, herb gardens that include a variety of plants can be almost pest-free. Pests' aversion to some odors is so powerful that many gardeners routinely plant selected herbs as companions to their vegetables and flowers, or place potted herbs among the plants they want to protect.

But pest problems can strike herbs. A 100-square-foot bed of nothing but basil will be irresistible to any Japanese beetles that happen along, for example, and hungry rose chafers often find patches of as few as six or seven basil plants growing together. Similarly, if you grow parsley in the same spot every year, you're giving carrot weevil populations a chance to build to damaging levels. See "Controlling Pest Problems" on page 54 for a list of the most common pests and recommended controls.

Your best protection against pests is to take these steps:

● Mix different herbs together in a bed.

● Grow your annual herbs in a different part of

HERBS AS PEST-REPELLING COMPANION PLANTS

The pest-repellent qualities of herbs are sometimes dismissed as "old gardeners' tales." But since many experienced gardeners, both old and young, swear by certain combinations, it makes sense to try them yourself. The following list contains some of the most widely recommended herbal pest repellents. Each of the herbs listed with a particular pest is reputed to repel that pest.

Pest	Repellent Herbs	Pest	Repellent Herbs
Ants	Tansy, wormwood	Imported cabbage moths	Anise hyssop, chives, dill, nasturtiums, pennyroyal, sage, southernwood, wormwood
Aphids	Chives, cilantro, fennel, peppermint, spearmint	Japanese beetles	Catnip, chives, garlic, tansy
Cabbage loopers	Anise hyssop, chives, nasturtiums, pennyroyal, sage, thyme	Mexican bean beetles	Rosemary, summer and winter savory
Carrot rust flies	Chives, rosemary, sage, wormwood	Slugs and snails	Fennel, garlic, rosemary
Codling moths	Wormwood	Spider mites	Cilantro
Colorado potato beetles	Catnip, cilantro, nasturtiums, tansy	Squash bugs	Catnip, nasturtiums, tansy
Cucumber beetles	Catnip, nasturtiums, rue	Tomato hornworms	Borage, dill, opal basil
Flea beetles	Rue, tansy, wormwood	Whiteflies	Nasturtiums, thyme, wormwood

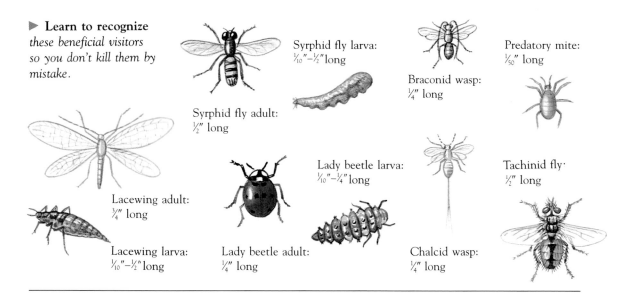

▶ **Learn to recognize** *these beneficial visitors so you don't kill them by mistake.*

Syrphid fly adult: ½" long

Syrphid fly larva: ¹⁄₁₀"–½" long

Braconid wasp: ¼" long

Predatory mite: ¹⁄₅₀" long

Lacewing adult: ¾" long

Lacewing larva: ¹⁄₁₀"–½" long

Lady beetle adult: ¼" long

Lady beetle larva: ¹⁄₁₀"–¼" long

Chalcid wasp: ¼" long

Tachinid fly· ½" long

the bed every year, and every four years, transplant your perennial herbs to different parts of the bed.

- Apply compost to add organic matter and encourage beneficial organisms.
- Weed, feed, water, mulch, and clean up conscientiously to maintain a healthy garden where pests have no place to hide.

YOUR ALLIES – THE BENEFICIAL INSECTS

Most insects in the herb garden have no direct effect on your plants. And only a few of the insects in your garden are pests. A handful of insects are actively beneficial, preying on or parasitizing garden pests. So before you squash that bug, check to be certain that it isn't one of your garden allies.

Many beneficial insects require a source of pollen or nectar during the adult phase of their lives. Some beneficials, such as lady beetles, are so large that they can feed on a variety of flowers in the garden. Others, such as the tiny parasitic wasps, must have tiny flowers.

Luckily, herb flowers provide the ideal foods for beneficial insects. If you're in the habit of pulling out herbs that have begun to flower because their leaves are past their prime, you may

want to consider the needs of these small but important allies and spare a few plants. Try to leave at least a few of the following flowers in your herb garden all summer long: caraway, chervil, cilantro, dill, mint, parsley, and yarrow.

DISEASES IN THE HERB GARDEN

Diseases are rarely a major problem in herb gardens. Commercial herb growers, with acres and acres of the same plant, do experience crop-threatening diseases, but in a home garden, there are usually so many different plants growing in a small space that disease organisms don't often build to damaging populations.

Exceptions to this rule occur, of course, so it's wise to practice preventive measures as much as possible. Prevention, rather than cure, is the most sensible way to deal with plant diseases. Plants don't fight off diseases with immune-system responses the way people do. Instead, their protection comes from basic good health and soils with high populations of beneficial microorganisms that prey on pathogenic ones. The garden environment and routine care play a part too. In crowded plantings where the humidity is quite high, fungi are likely to strike. Watering very late in the day can also stimulate an attack.

CONTROLLING PEST PROBLEMS

A healthy, well-tended herb garden that holds a variety of plants will avoid most common pest problems. Only occasionally will you need to try one of these effective organic controls

Pest	Herb Affected	Biological Controls	Physical Controls	Organic Sprays and Dusts	Cultural Controls
Aphid: $\frac{1}{12}''$–$\frac{1}{5}''$	Many, especially caraway, chervil, nasturtiums, oregano, parsley	Aphid midge (*Aphidoletes aphidomyza*), lacewings, lady beetles, parasitic wasps, syrphid flies	Squashing; hard spray of water	Insecticidal soap	Foil mulch; proper plant nutrition
Carrot weevil: $\frac{1}{5}''$	Parsley	Beneficial nematodes	Squashing		Crop rotation; compost (contains beneficial organisms that prey on this pest)
Cutworm: 2″	Most seedlings	Beneficial nematodes			Cardboard collars; insert 3 toothpicks into soil around plant stem to block cutworms
Earwig: $\frac{3}{4}''$	Angelica	Tachinid flies	Handpicking		Fall cleanup; avoid wood mulch
Japanese beetle: $\frac{1}{2}''$	Basil	Beneficial nematodes	Handpicking		Pheromone traps, set well away from garden
Leafminer: $\frac{1}{10}''$	Angelica, lovage, nasturtiums, oregano, sorrel		Remove and destroy all infested leaves		Cover plants with floating row cover
Mealybug: $\frac{1}{10}''$–$\frac{1}{4}''$	Rosemary	Lacewings, mealybug destroyer (*Cryptolaemus montrouzieri*)	Hard spray of water	Swab pests with alcohol; insecticidal soap	

Pest	Herb Affected	Biological Controls	Physical Controls	Organic Sprays and Dusts	Cultural Controls
Mint flea beetle: $\frac{1}{10}$"	Mints			Diatomaceous earth; lime dust	Cover young plants with floating row cover
Mite, spider: $\frac{1}{50}$"	Angelica, lemon verbena, mints, oregano, rosemary, sage, thyme	Lacewings, lady beetles, predatory mites	Spray of cold water; frequent misting	Insecticidal soap; sulfur	
Parsleyworm: 2" (swallowtail butterfly larvae)	Parsley	*Bacillus thuringiensis* (BT)	Handpicking		If you're willing to share your parsley with these caterpillars, you can enjoy butterflies in your herb garden later in the summer.
Rose chafer: $\frac{1}{2}$"	Basil		Handpicking		Crop rotation
Scale: $\frac{1}{10}$"–$\frac{1}{4}$"	Rosemary	Vidalia lady beetle		Swab pests with alcohol; insecticidal soap	
Slug: 3"	Many, especially basil, calendula, sage, violet		Handpicking; trap under boards; beer traps		Pull mulches away from plants in wet weather
Snail: 3"	Calendula		Handpicking; trap under boards; beer traps		Pull mulches away from plants in wet weather
Spittlebug: $\frac{1}{3}$"	Sage		Remove spittle (with insect)		Keep lawn and weeds mowed
Whitefly: $\frac{1}{12}$"	Lemon verbena, rosemary, scented geraniums	*Encarsia formosa*	Yellow sticky traps	Insecticidal soap; pyrethrins	

COMMON DISEASES IN THE HERB GARDEN

Disease	Plants Affected	Prevention and Controls	Disease	Plants Affected	Prevention and Controls
Anthracnose	Mints	Thin crowded plants, water early in the day, clean up old plant tissue in fall. If severe, dig out and destroy infected plants. Place new plants in a different spot. As a last resort, spray copper fungicide.	Leaf spot	Many, particularly lavender, nasturtiums, violets	Space plants appropriately. Remove all spotted leaves immediately and destroy. Wash hands and tools before moving to another spot.
Bacterial wilt	Nasturtiums, sage, scented geraniums	Do not plant where members of the tomato family have grown within 3 years. Prune off infected branches. If disease continues, dig and destroy plant.	Powdery mildew	Bee balm, calendula, cilantro, lemon balm, tarragon, yarrow	Thin herbs to increase air circulation. Compost tea sprays prevent attacks. Spray with superior oil and baking soda at the first sign of infection.
Botrytis blight	Rosemary, scented geraniums	Plant in well-drained soils, reduce humidity if possible, remove spent blossoms immediately. Compost tea often prevents infection.	Root rot	Many, particularly lavender, oregano, rosemary, sage, tarragon, thyme, winter savory	Wait until soils are sufficiently warm to plant or transplant. Plant in well-drained soils and avoid overwatering.
Crown rot	Angelica, parsley, violets	Reduce watering. If plant dies, remove all roots and soil and place new plants in a different location.			
Damping-off	Most seedlings	Reduce humidity around plants, increase air circulation if inside.	Rust	Bee balm, mints, yarrow	Do not overfertilize with nitrogen fertilizers. Reduce humidity. Pick off and destroy all infected leaves immediately.
Downy mildew	Calendula, cilantro, tarragon, violets	Remove infected leaves immediately. Clean up the garden thoroughly in fall. Compost tea sprays may prevent the mildew's attack.	Stem rot	Yarrow	Reduce humidity and do not overwater. Pull mulches back from plant stems. Compost tea sprays prevent infection.
Fusarium wilt	Basil	Buy certified disease-free seed. Rotate plantings, pull all diseased plants at the first sign of leaf spotting.	Verticillium wilt	Cilantro, mints, nasturtiums, sage	Resist planting or transplanting until weather is sufficiently warm. Rotate annuals. Clean up the garden thoroughly in fall.

Fortunately for gardeners, the techniques that make taking care of plants easier also help to prevent diseases. Appropriate spacing and weeding help to reduce humidity levels. Good soil drainage makes roots less susceptible to soil-dwelling disease organisms. A good, but not too rich, soil with enough nutrients strengthens the plants' ability to tolerate some diseases. Soil organic matter feeds beneficial predators. Locating plants where they will grow best, whether it's in bright light and dry soil or partial shade and moist conditions, also helps.

WHEN DISEASE THREATENS

If your plants do get a disease, the first step is proper identification. Good identification guides are listed in "Recommended Reading" on page 156. Your next step is to correct the conditions in your garden that led to the disease outbreak. Pay particular attention to all the elements that influence humidity around your plants – air movement, plant density, and watering patterns – because many of the most troublesome diseases strike only when humidity is high.

Some diseases are so localized that you can literally pluck them off the plant. Check "Common Diseases in the Herb Garden" opposite to learn if the particular disease your plant is hosting can be handled in this way. If so, remember to do this as soon as you notice problems. To avoid spreading fungal spores or bacteria to other leaves, put all the plucked leaves in a plastic bag and then throw them away. Be aware that you can carry fungi and bacteria from diseased plants to healthy ones on your tools, clothes, and shoes as you work in your garden. If you think you're dealing with a severe and potentially wide-spreading disease problem, it's worth the trouble to change your clothes and shoes and wash your tools thoroughly before going back out into the garden.

Several organic sprays are effective against diseases. Researchers are discovering that compost tea prevents many diseases from attacking.

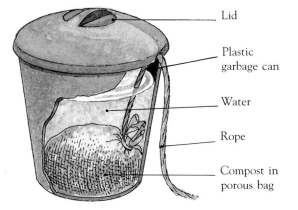

Lid

Plastic garbage can

Water

Rope

Compost in porous bag

▲ **Make compost tea** *with 1 part compost to 5 parts water. Let it soak for 1 to 2 weeks, then spray on foliage in early morning.*

To work well, this spray should be applied every two or three weeks from the beginning of the season through the fall.

Superior, or superfine, horticultural oil, mixed with baking soda, kills the powdery mildew fungus. Mix it as directed on the bottle and then add 4 teaspoons of baking soda to every gallon of solution. Spray this material on both sides of plant leaves.

Copper and sulfur fungicides also kill some disease organisms. However, they should be regarded as last-resort remedies. Even when sprayed correctly, they are strong enough to injure delicate plant tissues. Test by spraying a few leaves and watching them for several days to check for damage.

When you must spray, do it very early in the morning or on a cloudy day to avoid injuring leaves. Choose a still day, when wind is unlikely to cause any drift onto plants other than those you want to spray. Wear protective clothing and clean your clothes, shoes, and equipment properly when you're done. With a healthy, well-tended garden, you'll have little need to spray, but it's important to follow the proper precautions, no matter how harmless the material you're spraying might seem.

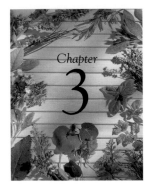

Chapter
3

USING AND ENJOYING YOUR HERBS

❧

HOMEGROWN HERBS *really shine in the kitchen. Fresh herbs, picked just moments before you use them, taste so good that you'll wonder how you ever managed without them. Once your herb garden is up and growing, you'll be amazed at the creativity it inspires at mealtimes. And seasoning your meals with fresh herbs is only the beginning. In addition to lots of ideas for using herbs straight from your garden, this chapter offers plenty of tips for preserving that just-picked flavor in dried or frozen herbs. You'll find out which storage techniques work best for each herb you grow, as well as how to use those herbs once they're dried or frozen. Herb-flavored vinegars and oils are another way to preserve your herbs for year-round use, and they make lovely gifts from your garden, too. Or try your hand at making herb teas, jellies, salads, breads, and honeys — you'll find recipes for all these delights and more in the pages ahead.*

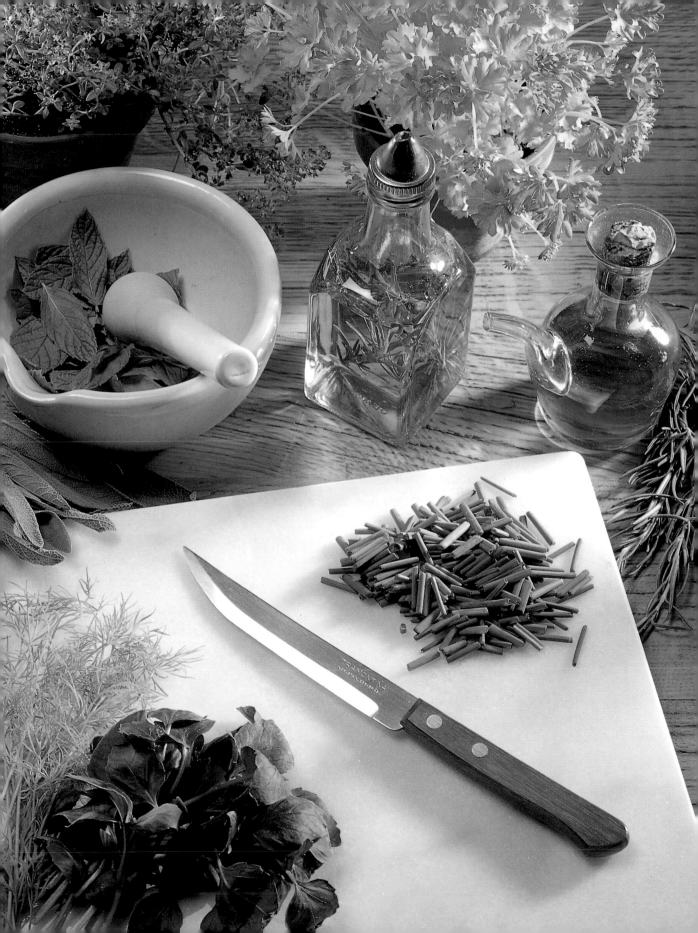

Harvesting Your Herbs

Imagine the taste of homegrown tomatoes seasoned with your own freshly picked basil. Picture delighting your friends with custom-made teas or potpourris made from herbs you've grown yourself.

Once your herb garden gets growing, you can harvest from it nearly every day if you like. After all, no dinner is complete without a few herbs to season it, so you may want to visit the garden daily to snip a little of this or a lot of that. Obviously, the best time to harvest herbs for immediate use is when you need them. But if you're gathering herbs to dry or freeze for future use, you'll want to be sure to pick them when flavors are at their peak.

PICKING FOR PEAK FLAVOR
AND FRAGRANCE

To enjoy the fullest fragrances and flavors from herb leaves, harvest young leaves from your herbs before they bloom. You'll get better-tasting herbs if you pick the young leaves several times a season, rather than waiting until the whole plant is nearly mature. Pick herb flowers when they're not quite in full bloom or on the very day when they first open their petals.

The concentration of the oils that give herbs their wonderful aromas and flavors is strongest when the plant is still cool. That's why morning is the best time to harvest herb leaves or flowers, no matter whether you'll use them in dried arrangements, preserve them, or add them to your evening meal. Flowers are more likely to hold their shape and retain their petals if you pick them before they warm up.

HARVESTING BY THE MOON

Many gardeners plant and harvest by moon phases and signs. They say herbs harvested on a moon calendar retain more nutrients and have improved keeping qualities. Though the success of your herb garden won't rest on this technique alone, it can't hurt to try it. Pick your herbs in the morning as usual, but aim for the dates when the moon is at an auspicious phase. Consult a moon calender (see "Recommended Reading" on page 156) to find exactly when the time is right to pick.

Plant Part	Moon Indicators
Roots	Waxing moon, in Aries, Leo, Sagittarius, Gemini, or Aquarius
Seeds	Just after full moon, in Leo, Sagittarius, Gemini, or Aquarius
Leaves and flowers for drying	Waning moon, in Aries, Leo, Sagittarius, Gemini, or Aquarius
Leaves for freezing	Waxing moon, in Scorpio, Pisces, Cancer, Libra, or Taurus

TO RINSE OR NOT TO RINSE?

One of the pleasures of gardening organically is that you can eat your food without worrying about washing it. You can pop a strawberry into your mouth or nibble a sprig of peppermint as you stroll through the garden. There are no chemical residues to wash off. Many organic gardeners rinse their herbs only as needed to remove splashed-on soil, or to wash off any insects that might be hiding in the leaves.

Whether or not you wash your herbs before using them also depends on how soon you want to eat them. If you're picking them to put in tonight's salad, the choice is up to you. But if you plan to store them for a few days, hold off on washing until you're ready to use them, unless you're picking parsley. Parsley is one herb that does benefit from a plunge into cool water soon after picking; it stays fresh longer and doesn't wilt. Shake off the extra water before storing.

A FRESH SUPPLY OF LEAVES AND FLOWERS

Putting aside a day or two's supply of fresh herbs is remarkably easy. Just pop newly picked leaves or flowers into an open plastic bag and store them in the refrigerator. Don't seal or tie the bag closed; a bit of air will help keep the herbs fresh. Perforated plastic vegetable storage bags are perfect for holding fresh herbs. Rinse, if you like, just before using. Fresh-picked leaves and flowers can rot or turn moldy if you store them in moist conditions.

COLLECTING TASTY SEEDS

Let seeds of herbs such as dill, caraway, and anise ripen on the plant to reach their full flavor and fragrance. Most herbs drop their seeds when they're ripe, so you'll want to keep an eye on your plants to catch the seeds before they fall. When you notice seedpods plumping up or exposed seeds beginning to turn brown, that means they'll soon be ripe and ready. When the seeds are ripe, bend the stalk toward the ground and shake the seeds into a paper bag.

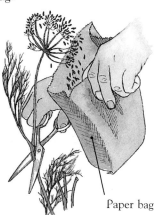

▶ **Ripe seeds** *may fall to the ground when you're harvesting. Hold a paper bag where it will catch falling seeds as you cut.*

Paper bag

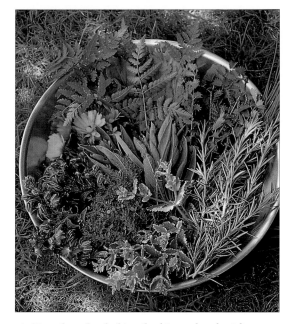

▲ **Develop the habit** *of taking a bowl with you when you visit the herb garden – a scent or flavor might inspire the perfect dinner.*

Ripening is a gradual process. If you're not sure of your timing, add the insurance of a paper bag. When you notice signs of ripening, enclose the seed head in a small paper bag and close it around the stem with a rubber band or twist tie. When you can hear seeds rattle when you shake the stem, snip the stem several inches below the bag to harvest the entire seed head.

DIGGING UP ROOTS

Be patient if you plan to harvest the roots of herbs such as angelica or comfrey. You'll get more for your efforts if you wait until the plants are at least two years old before you dig their roots. Even two-year-old roots of fibrous-rooted valerian will seem spindly, but rest assured that they're sufficiently potent.

Dig roots in the fall, after the herb's leaves have changed color or dropped. Scrub the roots, then cut them into 2-inch-long pieces for drying. (See page 62 for more on drying herbs.)

Drying Herbs

Drying is one of the simplest and most convenient ways to preserve your herbs' leaves and flowers. It's so easy to dry large amounts that you can keep a full winter's supply for yourself and still have plenty left for gift giving.

Most people use one of three drying methods – air drying by hanging the herbs, air drying on elevated screens, or drying in a dehydrator. Your choice of method depends as much on the eventual use you'll make of the herb as on its particular characteristics. Turn to the Directory, beginning on page 98, to find the best drying techniques to use for each herb you want to dry.

HANGING TO DRY

Hang drying is an excellent way to preserve herbs, especially in large quantities. You'll need a well-ventilated, dark, dry location to hang your herbs in. Your attic could be ideal (cover any windows to block the light), or perhaps you have a spare room that fits the bill.

Gather herbs for hang drying early in the day. Don't bother washing them off unless they are muddy. If you must rinse the herbs, let the surface moisture evaporate completely before you bunch them to hang. Spread the rinsed herbs on a slatted wooden drain rack, available at kitchen supply stores, so air can circulate and speed drying. Tie small bunches of herbs with twist ties, rubber bands, or elastic thread and hang them so that air can circulate freely around them.

If you're drying culinary herbs, enclose the bunches in small paper bags to keep the herbs from getting dusty while they dry. They'll take a little longer to dry this way – up to three weeks in good, well-ventilated conditions – but they'll stay as clean as the day you picked them. If your drying area is somewhat humid, use cheesecloth around the herbs instead of paper bags. Cheesecloth's open weave allows air to circulate around the herbs but still traps most of the dust.

Hang the bunches at least a foot from the wall and leave at least 6 inches between bunches. If you have only a few bunches to dry, an expandable laundry rack makes a handy and portable holder. If you're drying in quantity, you may want to make a more permanent arrangement. Screw small hooks into the ceiling at 3- to 4-foot intervals in rows across the room, and run strings

▲ **Bunches of herbs** *are decorative as they dry, long before they're used in arrangements.*

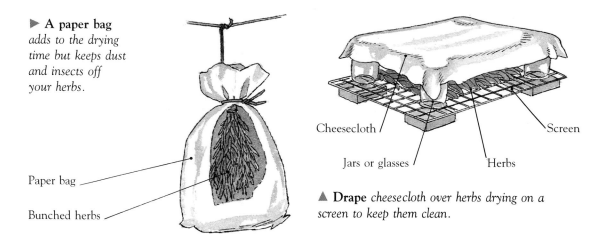

► **A paper bag** *adds to the drying time but keeps dust and insects off your herbs.*

Paper bag

Bunched herbs

Cheesecloth

Jars or glasses

Herbs

Screen

▲ **Drape** *cheesecloth over herbs drying on a screen to keep them clean.*

down each row of hooks. Tie the bunches of herbs to these strings.

Most herbs dry in about two weeks when hung in well-ventilated, dry, dark conditions. When they are completely dry, they'll feel crackly crisp to the touch. Either use them immediately or store them for later use. Because nearly all the water's been removed from them, dried herb flavors are more concentrated than fresh herbs. Reduce the amount you put in your recipes to one-half to one-third as much as you'd add if using fresh herbs.

When your culinary herbs are dried, strip the leaves from their stems and store in tightly closed bottles or jars in a dark cupboard. To store dried bunches of decorative herbs, wrap each bunch in tissue paper to protect it from damage. Lay the wrapped bunches flat in large cardboard boxes, and store the boxes in a dark, dry place until you're ready to use the herbs.

DRYING SEEDS

It's important to dry ripened herb seeds before you store them. If you don't already have the seed heads bagged, put them in roomy paper bags to finish drying after harvest. Fully ripe seeds will take only a week or two to drop from the seed head into the bottom of the bag, depending on their maturity and the humidity of your drying

room – the drier the air, the quicker they'll dry. After the seeds have dropped, pour them into a glass jar. If the air is humid, close the jar tightly; if it's dry, lay a piece of cheesecloth over the top of the jar's mouth. Each day for several days afterward, pour the seeds from their storage jar into another clean, dry jar. To see if they're dry, test the seeds occasionally by pushing your fingernail into one or two of them. When the seeds are hard, they're dry. Pour them into the jars you'll use to store them over the winter.

DRYING ON SCREENS AND DEHYDRATORS

Elevated screens are practical when you are drying very small material, such as tiny leaves, calendula petals, or chamomile flowers, that would otherwise be hard to handle. You can also use them for drying whole flowers or flower sprays in an open form.

Dehydrators are the answer if the humidity in your house is too high for successful air drying. They're also useful for herbs like parsley that lose much of their color and flavor when air dried, and they're great for drying pieces of roots. Leaves and flowers take only a day or two to dry in a dehydrator, while roots dry in about three days. When you dry small-leaved herbs, such as thyme, line each dehydrator tray with cheesecloth to keep the leaves from falling through.

Freezing Culinary Herbs

Freezing captures the full flavor of most herb leaves. If you don't have room for many herb plants in your indoor winter garden, freeze the others for a taste that's almost as good as fresh. Freezing is also an excellent way to preserve herbs like basil that lose or change flavor when dried.

If you're freezing small quantities, or if you pack the freezer bags lightly, freezing herbs is a breeze. Just chop the herbs, slip them into a freezer bag, label, and toss in the freezer. When you're ready to use them, simply break off as much as you need.

If you're freezing large quantities of herbs, however, or if you want to put more than a thin layer of chopped herbs in your freezer bags, it's better to freeze the leaves separately. Spread them out on a baking sheet and put them in the freezer. Once they're frozen, pour them off the baking sheet into bags for more efficient storage. This way the chopped pieces remain separate, so you can take out exactly what you need without having to chip away at a frozen block of leaves.

SPECIAL PREPARATIONS

Most herbs contain so much oil that they don't need to be blanched before being frozen. Basil and lovage are the only exceptions to this general rule. Both these herbs retain better color and flavor when you blanch them before freezing. Before you pack basil or lovage for the freezer, blanch them for about a minute, then cool in ice-cold water and dry on paper towels.

If you're freezing herbs to use mainly in soups or stews, here's a neat trick to combine blanching with preparation for the freezer. Pack your chopped up herbs in ice cube trays, then cover them with water and freeze. If you use boiling water to fill the trays, you'll blanch your herbs before freezing, without the separate step. Once the herbal cubes are frozen, you can pop them out of the trays and into freezer bags for storage. These cubes are handy for adding fresh-herb flavor to a simmering pot of soup.

If you'd rather skip the blanching altogether, you can also freeze basil, lovage, and most other herbs in oil, as described in "Freezing in Oil Cubes" opposite.

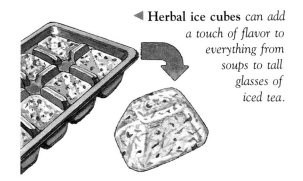

◀ **Herbal ice cubes** *can add a touch of flavor to everything from soups to tall glasses of iced tea.*

FREEZE THESE HERBS

Some herbs, including those listed below, lose their flavor when they are dried. But instead of giving them up for the winter, freeze them. Herbs that aren't on the following list can be frozen, too. Try freezing some bags filled with herbal combinations, such as the *fines herbes* – chervil, chives, parsley, and tarragon – that include some herbs that don't dry well.

Basil	Fennel
Chervil	Lovage
Chives	Parsley
Cilantro	Sweet cicely

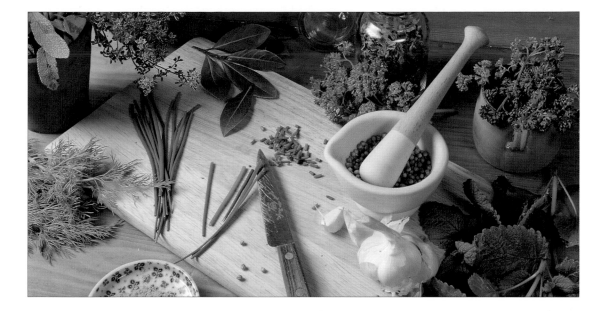

If you don't use the stems of your herbs in cooking, strip off the leaves before you freeze them and include only leaves in your freezer bag. For example, you'll want to remove basil leaves from the stems before blanching. On the other hand, the stems of parsley and cilantro have as much flavor as the leaves, so you'll want to freeze the whole sprigs. If your frozen herbs include stems mince the stems for cooking while they are still half-frozen. Frozen herbs aren't as concentrated as dried herbs because they still contain a lot of water. When you thaw them for use in a recipe calling for dried herbs, measure your frozen herbs as if they were fresh. Begin by using about three times as much as the recipe suggests for dried herbs. Taste as you cook to decide whether this is enough. If not, add more.

Keep experimenting with frozen herbs to discover the packing systems that work best for you. It's tremendously satisfying to reach into the freezer and find the perfect seasoning for whatever you're making.

FREEZING IN OIL CUBES

Frozen cilantro is far tastier than dried, but to get the maximum flavor from this herb, you'll want

▲ **Preparing herbs** *for freezing is surprisingly fast and simple. Begin by mincing up a few of your favorites and stowing them in the freezer. Thaw frozen herbs as needed for cooking. Before long, you'll have a supply of herbs to see you through the winter.*

to freeze it in oil. Mince the cilantro finely in a food processor, and then add olive oil until the mixture is a smooth paste. Pack the paste in small plastic bags or in an ice cube tray. When the small bags or cubes are frozen, put the frozen paste in a larger storage container or plastic bag, and label.

You can also freeze basil and lovage in oil. With this method, there's no need to blanch the herbs first. Prepare them as described above for cilantro, using olive oil with basil and canola oil with lovage. Lovage tastes better with canola oil's lighter flavor. Choose oils for freezing that will complement the flavor of your herbs and any recipes you plan to use the herbs in. Although basil is typically frozen in olive oil, you can preserve it in lighter oils, like canola or safflower, to avoid olive oil's more pronounced flavor.

Herbal Seasonings

Herbs transform ordinary meals into flavorful delights. Even if you already cook with herbs, a backyard herb garden can inspire you to experiment with the unfamiliar and discover new ways to use old favorites. Before long, you'll find yourself mixing sweet cicely into the pancake batter and stirring snips of savory into the bean soup.

You can make herbal seasonings fresh from the garden or from your stock of dried and frozen herbs. Keep in mind that dried herbs pack a more intense punch than fresh or frozen herbs. If you're using fresh or frozen herbs, you'll generally use about half to two-thirds more than if you're using dried herbs.

During the summer, for example, you might make a seasoned butter by mixing 1 teaspoon each of freshly picked marjoram, thyme, and rosemary and ¼ teaspoon each of fresh basil and sage into ½ cup of unsalted butter. In the winter, you can still make this spread by substituting your own dried herbs and decreasing the quantities by one-half to one-third. (Incidentally, even though basil changes flavor somewhat when it is dried, it still adds a wonderful taste to many recipes, from herbed butters to cooked sauces.)

MAKING READY-MADE HERBAL BLENDS

Already-mixed combinations of dried or frozen herbs are the key to speeding up your meal prep time. You can use them all through the year, whenever the time you have for cooking is short. A pinch or two from a jar of dried basil, oregano, rosemary, and thyme, for example, can give an instant lift to a quick pasta meal or pizza. A dried mixture of the lemon-flavored herbs – lemon balm, lemon basil, lemongrass leaves, lemon thyme, and lemon verbena – saves time when you're preparing fish or making a sauce for chicken. Frozen cubes of mixed basil, chives, cilantro, and parsley enliven the flavor of a chili when added just before serving.

Experiment during the summer with combination seasonings by drying small batches of the herbs you use most frequently and mixing them together in the proportions in which you use them. You'll soon discover which jars you reach for most often, and then you'll still have plenty of time to harvest, dry, and mix a pint or so of your favorites to give you that wonderful flavor through the winter.

FINES HERBES

1 Tbsp. chervil
1 Tbsp. parsley

1 Tbsp. chives
1 Tbsp. tarragon

Mince herbs finely and sprinkle over your dish – omelet, fish, or poultry – just before serving. Traditionally, *fines herbes* should contain equal measures, but you can vary it according to your dish.

COOKING WITH DRIED AND FROZEN HERBS

Your own dried herbs always taste much better than anything you can buy in a store. For one thing, they're freshly made. A few kitchen tricks can enhance their flavor too. A savory beginning is to add dried herbs to oil, turn the heat to low, and stir them for a few minutes before going on with the recipe. When using dried herbs in salad dressings or other cold preparations, mix and let it set at room temperature for an hour or so before serving, to bring out the flavor. (See page 68 for more about salads.) Seeds hide their flavor under a hard coat. To release their full aroma and taste, heat dried seeds in a skillet before adding them to a cooked dish, or crush them in a mortar and pestle just before using.

Frozen herbs add rich flavor to soups, stews, and sauces, and in most cases you can just toss them into the pot while it's simmering. But keep in mind that frozen herbs contain water. If you're planning to add frozen herbs to biscuit doughs or herb butters, where extra moisture could cause problems, you'll want to thaw the herbs first and drain off the water. When you are using frozen herbs in a thickened sauce, thaw the herbs and drain them before adding them to the sauce, so the extra water doesn't dilute it. Or add frozen herbs at the very end of the cooking time and then cook down the sauce over very low heat.

▶ **Herbal butters** *are a snap to make and can add wonderful flavors to your meals. Choose herbs to complement your dish, mince them finely, and mix them into softened butter.*

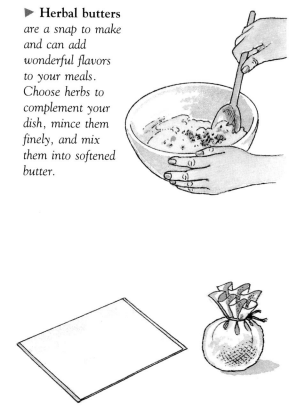

▲ ***Bouquet garni*** *starts with a bay leaf, thyme, and parsley; add other herbs as desired.*

AVOCADO SALAD

2 Tbsp. lemon juice
1 Tbsp. olive oil
Salt and pepper

2 ripe avocados
2 Tbsp. chopped chervil

Mix the lemon juice and olive oil together, add salt and pepper, and place in a bowl. Peel and slice the avocado into the lemon juice mixture, covering pieces thoroughly. Chill for an hour. Sprinkle on chervil just before serving.

Dressing Up Salads

Salads have become a regular part of American meals — sometimes the salad is the meal — and they are becoming more interesting too. Instead of the old standard iceberg lettuce, good restaurants and home cooks are more likely to serve a salad of interesting greens, such as arugula and radicchio, several kinds of lettuce, and a variety of herbs and flowers.

You can buy convenient bagged salad mixes that combine lettuce, greens, and herbs, or you can buy basic salad greens and dress them up yourself with additions from your herb garden. A good herb garden gives you the luxury of being able to serve salads with as many exotic ingredients as you want. Of course, if you grow the salad greens too, your meal will be even fresher and better tasting.

DINING ON DELECTABLE BLOSSOMS

Edible flowers are one of the most delightful additions to a salad of greens or fruits. You can't tell what a flower tastes like by looking at it, so take a little nibble of your edible blossoms to learn how they taste. Nasturtium blossoms, for example, have a sharp, peppery bite. Borage flowers taste of cucumbers, violets are almost sweet, bee balm florets are minty, chive florets are spicy-oniony, and garlic chives flower heads are slightly garlicky.

Flowers lose quality quickly when they are wet, so it's best not to wash them when you harvest. Besides, there's an easier way to free your flowers of any lurking insects. Put the blossoms into a plastic bag. Blow into the bag to inflate it and secure it with a twist tie. Set the bag in the refrigerator for at least half an hour. If there were any flying insects inside the flowers, they will be clinging to the bag when you remove it. Other insects will have dropped to the bottom of the bag. If you still want to wash the flowers, wait until the last minute before serving.

COMBINING HERBS WITH IMAGINATION

Cooking has become more imaginative, thanks to the blossoming of American cuisine. New combinations are turning up all the time. For an herb gardener, this is a boon. Your herbs can add intriguing aromas and flavors, or they can help to marry the flavors of other ingredients. Try making a luncheon salad of a cubed half cantaloupe, 2 medium tomatoes cut into wedges, and 1 grated cucumber, dressed with 1 cup of plain yogurt to which you've added ½ to ¾ cup finely minced spearmint or peppermint. Or make a delightfully spicy salad that's half lettuce and half nasturtium blossoms. Dress this with olive oil, lemon juice, and 1 tablespoon or more of chervil.

Some herbs do great things in fruit salads. Angelica, anise, bee balm flowers, hyssop, lemon balm, mints, and sweet cicely are all pleasant surprises when combined with fruits. Try sweet cicely in a salad to which you want to give a little sweetness without using sugar. Anise and hyssop seeds give apple and pear salads a richer taste. Lemon balm, bee balm flowers, and mints are particularly good with citrus fruits.

Main dish salads benefit from the addition of herbs, too. Try making a cold rice or bulgur salad by mixing the cooked grain with finely diced vegetables, some cold cooked chick-peas or black beans, cubed cheese, and an herbed oil and vinegar salad dressing.

Basic Herbed Italian Dressing

¾ cup olive oil
¼ cup vinegar (can be an herbal vinegar)

2 Tbsp. minced fresh herbs of your choice

Mix oil and vinegar in a jar with a tight-fitting lid. Shake vigorously. Add minced herbs to the dressing. Let sit for an hour at room temperature. Shake again before serving.

Herb and Yogurt Dressing

1 cup plain acidophilus yogurt
½ cup extra-virgin olive oil
½ cup tarragon vinegar
Salt

Pepper
Minced fresh chives, dill, lemon balm, parsley, sage, and spearmint, to taste
Few drops of maple syrup

Shake yogurt, oil, and vinegar together in a jar. Add salt, pepper, minced herbs, and maple syrup. Shake again before serving.

Green Mayonnaise

1 egg yolk
1 cup extra-virgin olive oil
1 Tbsp. wine vinegar
2 Tbsp. finely minced fresh parsley

2 Tbsp. finely minced fresh chervil or other herbs (basil, rosemary, thyme)

Beat egg yolk till it becomes slightly pale in color. Drop by drop, while you are still beating, add ¾ cup olive oil. Still beating, add vinegar. Continue beating while you add the final ¼ cup olive oil. Add parsley and other herbs to taste.

Try *these classic herbal dressings on your salads and see what a difference they make. When possible, use fresh herbs rather than dried to enjoy the fullest flavors.*

Brewing Herbal Vinegars

Herbal vinegars perk up salads and other dishes with a flavor all their own. They're easy to prepare, beautiful to look at, and fun to collect. And they make great gifts from the garden.

The flavor of an herbal vinegar is deeper and richer than the flavor of a vinegar to which dried herbs have been added before serving. The acid in the vinegar draws out the essential oils in the herbs, giving the final product a wonderful, complex mix of flavors. You can use an herbal vinegar in any recipe that calls for vinegar and in many recipes to which you add lemon. A dash of tarragon vinegar in deviled eggs or macaroni and cheese, for example, adds a subtle flavor and also gives a taste that seems fresh and clean. A few teaspoons of a parsley-rosemary-sage red wine vinegar brings out the flavors in a beef stew.

Because herbal vinegars taste so strongly of whatever herb they're made with, they make good table condiments. A sprinkling of chive-flower vinegar perks up any of the greens in the cabbage family – kale, mustard, collards – and it does something wonderful to raw cabbage salads. Once you have a shelf of richly flavored vinegars, you'll be inspired to create many more interesting ways to use them.

The procedure for making any herbal vinegar is the same, no matter what herb or combination of herbs you're using. All you need are some herbs or herb flowers, vinegar, glass jars, and a glass or stainless steel saucepan.

Use only top-quality herbs, picked at the peak of their flavor. (See pages 60 and 99 for guidelines on when to pick.) The vinegars you buy to

A SAMPLING OF HERBAL VINEGARS

Herbal vinegars add bright, fresh flavors to salads and sauces, and they make great, healthful condiments for all sorts of foods. Experiment with different herbs and herb combinations, as well as with different vinegars, to create the signature seasonings for your favorite dishes. When you find an herbal vinegar you especially like, be sure to prepare a few extra bottles – herbal vinegars make lovely gifts from your garden.

Herb or Herbal Combination	Type of Vinegar	Uses for Finished Herbal Vinegar
Chive flowers	White wine	Salads, marinades, sauces
Tarragon	White wine	Salads; sauces for fish, chicken, eggs
Chive flowers, savory*	White wine or cider	Cold bean salad
Dill, garlic-chive flowers, nasturtiums*	White wine or cider	Salads, cooked greens or snap beans
Mints, sweet cicely seeds*	White wine	Fruit salads, cooked peas
Parsley, rosemary, sage*	Red wine	Potato salad, grain or tofu salads

*Combine these herbs in equal parts.

combine with your herbs should be top quality too. Wine vinegars, white or red, are almost always preferable to cider vinegar, although cider vinegar does complement some of the annual herbs like summer savory and dill. You can also use rice vinegar, particularly when you are using a very delicately flavored herb such as chervil.

MAKING HERBAL VINEGAR

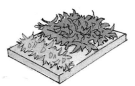

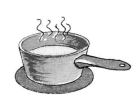

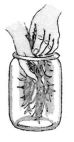

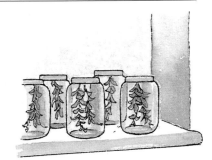

1 *Begin making an herbal vinegar by mincing the herbs that will flavor it.*

2 *Heat the vinegar until it is warm but not boiling.*

3 *Bruise the herbs as you add them to the jar.*

4 *Steep the vinegar for two weeks, strain, and rebottle.*

Vinegar reacts with many metals, especially aluminum. Heat the vinegar in either a glass or stainless steel saucepan to prevent it from picking up an off flavor. Always steep your herbal vinegars in glass jars. Not only do you want the light to penetrate the jar while the vinegar is brewing, you also want to safeguard the flavor. While it might seem practical to make vinegars in standard canning jars, the vinegar will eventually corrode the metal lids and rims. Old-fashioned canning jars with rubber rings and glass lids with wire bails will work, but it's hard to find them anywhere unless you hit a particularly good yard sale. Fortunately, one source of good steeping containers is available in any neighborhood. Institutional kitchens, including restaurants and school cafeterias, usually have gallon mayonnaise jars, with plastic lids, that they're happy to save for you. Unless you're going into business with herbal vinegars, four or five of these jars can see you through a season of vinegar making.

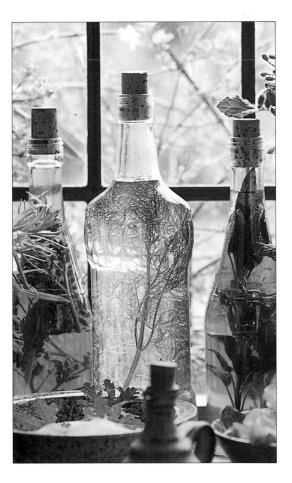

▶ **Herbal vinegars** *delight the eyes as well as the palate. To make them even lovelier, add a few fresh herb sprigs when you bottle the vinegar.*

Herb-Flavored Oils

Herbal oils are another great way to use your bountiful herb harvest. Like herbal vinegars, herb-flavored oils taste quite different than oil into which you've mixed some dried or fresh herbs. The herbal flavor is stronger and present in every bite. You can use these oils in salad or vegetable dressings, marinades, and sauces.

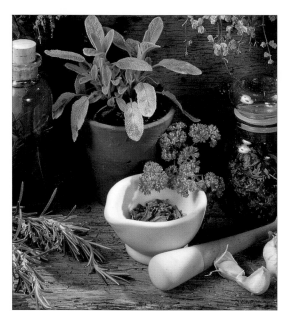

▲ **Crush herbs** *before soaking them in an oil when preparing them for a pesto or for an herb-flavored oil for freezing.*

SAFETY FIRST

Oils have been used as preservatives for many thousands of years, but despite this long history, there are some crucial safety factors to keep in mind. In recent years, food scientists have been advising people to take safety measures when making flavored oils to avoid the risk of botulism. Botulism is a toxin produced by the bacterium *Clostridium botulinum*, found in soil, water, and air. This bacterium grows readily when placed in an environment, such as oil, that lacks oxygen.

If you are adding garlic (or chile peppers or other vegetables) to your oil, soak it in vinegar for 8 to 24 hours before adding it to the oil. The vinegar acidifies the garlic and curtails bacterial growth. Strain the garlic from the vinegar and place it in a sterile container, then cover with oil and refrigerate. Use the oil within three weeks. To be safe, store all herb-and-oil combinations in the refrigerator and use them promptly.

Freezing is another way to safely store your herb-oil mixtures. Freeze them in small packets for use during the winter. Start by finely chopping about 2 cups of herbs. Mix them with about ¼ cup of the oil of your choice. Spoon the mixture into small plastic bags, label, and freeze. To use a packet, let it thaw at room temperature.

To flavor oil for immediate use, heat the oil in a small saucepan and add chopped herbs and other seasonings, such as garlic, to the oil.

HERBS IN OIL

Preserve these herbs in oil to bring new flavors to your main dishes. Try mixing herbs with complementary flavors to create a flavorful cooking oil blend.

Basil	Oregano
Chervil	Parsley
Chives	Rosemary
Coriander	Sage
Dill	Tarragon
Fennel	Thyme
Lemon verbena	

PESTO

3 cups packed fresh basil
  leaves
½ to ¾ cup packed fresh
  parsley
¼ cup grated Parmesan or
  Romano cheese

½ cup nuts (pine nuts,
  walnuts, or cashews)
½ cup olive oil
3 to 6 cloves garlic
Dash of black pepper

Place all ingredients in a blender or food processor and mix until smooth. Toss with hot pasta.

VARIATION: Almost any aromatic herb can be used in a pesto instead of the basil.

CHOOSING THE OIL

Extra-virgin olive oil complements the flavor of the herbs we consider "Mediterranean" – basil, oregano, and thyme. Herbs such as chives, parsley, and rosemary also have intense flavors that blend well with olive oil.

Some foods and recipes require a lighter, less dominant oil. Asian cuisine, for example, tastes best when peanut or canola oil is used. To give yourself flexibility later in the year, preserve herbs that you expect to use in Asian cooking in either one of these oils. Remember to label packets with a note on both the herb and the oil used. Tarragon and chervil benefit from being preserved in a lighter oil like canola or safflower.

The citrusy flavors of lemon thyme and lemon verbena taste wonderful when mixed with walnut oil. This herbal oil mixture is particularly good when used in a dressing for leafy green salads.

Remember that the oil you choose is a matter of taste. If olive oil's heavy flavor doesn't suit your palate or the dishes you're cooking, or for maximum flexibility, choose a light, flavorless oil like safflower or canola.

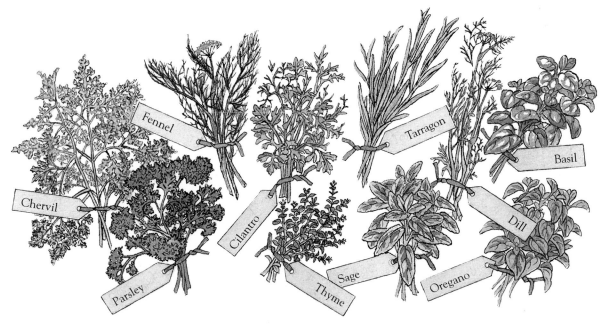

Making Herb Teas

It's no wonder herb teas are so popular. They taste great, have no calories or caffeine, and can be enjoyed hot or iced. Once found only in health food stores, herb teas have become a standard item in most groceries and a regular menu feature in many restaurants.

Using the herbs you grow in your garden, you'll find it's fun and easy to create your own custom herb tea blend. Homemade herb tea has a fresh flavor you won't find in a package, and it makes a great gift that will delight your family and friends.

Just as homegrown fruits and vegetables taste many times better than those you can buy, homemade herb teas have a fresher, cleaner taste than their commercial counterparts. They brew up into wonderfully fragrant, flavorful teas. And because you grow your herbs organically and dry them naturally, you can enjoy your homemade teas knowing they're made with wholesome ingredients that are free of pesticide residues.

CHOOSING A DELIGHTFUL MIX OF FLAVORS

A sampling of mints, a patch of chamomile, and four to six lemon balm plants make a good beginning for your tea garden. These plants are the basics. They make fine teas all by themselves, and they're even better when you combine them with other delightful flavors.

When choosing herbs for tea, let your nose guide you as you wander through the garden. Mints make a good base flavor. The lemon-flavored herbs – lemon balm, lemon thyme, and lemon verbena – add some sparkle to the basic tea. Borage leaves supply a cooling note, while

anise gives a hint of licorice. If you want to make your basic green-colored teas more colorful, try bee balm. The dried flowers, in shades of red, pink, and purple, make a colorful cupful.

Add a delicate sweetness to the brew with leaves of rose geranium or sweet cicely. Taste your tea before adding honey to it – the natural sweetenings of these herbs may be all you need.

To find out which herbs are good candidates for the teapot, see "Herbs at a Glance" on pages 9–12 and the Directory listings on pages 100–153 for specific herbs.

FRESH OR DRIED?

You can make your teas from either fresh or dried herbs – both will yield fine-flavored teas. Jars of dried herbs give you a taste of summer all through the cold seasons. If you dry a broad selection of herbs, you can have as much variety in January as

---

TEAS TO TRY

Many of your favorite herbs will make excellent tea on their own with no added ingredients. But it's fun to make up herb tea blends, since a combination of herbs has a more complex flavor than a single herb alone. Begin by experimenting with the following blends, then let your imagination suggest others.

- Anise, chamomile, and bee balm
- Betony and lavender flowers
- Borage flowers with lemon verbena and lemon balm
- Chamomile and spearmint or apple mint
- Chamomile and valerian
- Lemon verbena, lemongrass, and lemon thyme
- Scented geranium and chocolate mint
- Scented geranium and lemongrass
- Spearmint and peppermint

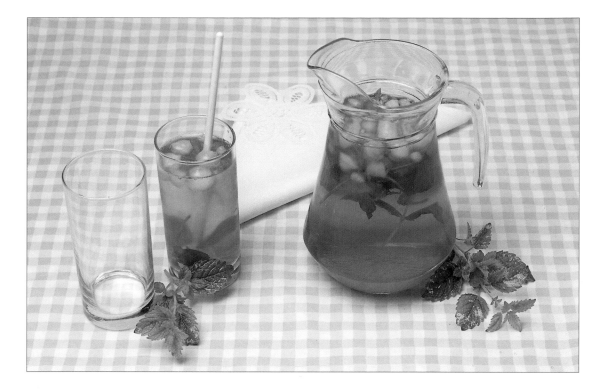

▲ **Homegrown tea herbs** *are one of the best reasons for starting an herb garden. Not only will you enjoy having great tea through the year, you can also mix blends for gifts.*

you enjoy in July. (You'll find instructions for drying your herbs for future use in "Drying Herbs" on page 62.) When it comes time to make tea, start with a teaspoon or so of dried herbs per cup of water, plus 1 to 2 teaspoons of herbs to flavor the pot. Tea making isn't an exact science – you may need to adjust the amount of herbs you use to get your tea to the strength you like.

During the summer, when your backyard herbs are growing green and strong, put on the kettle and take a trip through the garden. Pick at least 2 tablespoons of fresh herbs for every cup of tea, plus a tablespoon or two for the pot. Fresh herbs have more water in their leaves than dried ones, so you'll need to use larger amounts of them in tea making, just as you do in cooking.

BREWING THE PERFECT POT OF TEA

To let the full, delicate flavor of your herbal teas shine through, steep them in a glass or ceramic teapot. Don't use metal teapots; even stainless steel can change the flavor of your tea. Here's how to brew the perfect pot of tea:

1 Put a kettle of water on to boil for making the tea.

2 In the meantime, preheat your teapot. Fill the empty pot with hot water and let it sit for a few minutes.

3 Just before the tea water comes to a boil, pour out the heating water in the teapot, add your herbs to the pot, and bruise them with a wooden spoon to release the flavors.

4 When the kettle of water just begins to boil, pour it into the teapot.

5 Cover and let the tea steep for about five minutes before serving. If you aren't drinking the whole pot right away, strain out the herbs so the brew doesn't get too strong.

Herbal Jellies and Honeys

What could be nicer than herbal jelly on a morning biscuit? Perhaps herbal honey on a muffin. Whatever your choice, jelly or honey, growing your own herbs is the perfect inspiration for making some of these sweet treats.

DELICIOUSLY DIFFERENT HERBAL JELLY

Herbal jellies are particularly easy to make. If you've ever made fruit jellies, you know that much of the work involves simmering the fruit to extract its juice. Herbal jellies work another way: Most recipes only require you to make a very strong tea, or infusion, from the herb leaves. The infusion carries the flavor of the herb, just as juice carries the flavor of fruit. Because herb leaves lack pectin, the substance that thickens jellies, you'll have to add pectin to all herbal jellies.

SINFULLY SWEET HERBAL HONEY

Herb-flavored honey can be divine. Mint honey is probably the best-known herbal honey, but herb gardeners have the luxury of being able to experiment with more exotic flavors. Lavender and lemon verbena make spectacular honeys, for example, while anise seed, coriander, fennel seed, marjoram, rosemary, rose-scented geranium, sage, thyme, and violet all lend distinctive flavors to a pot of honey.

STEP-BY-STEP HERBAL HONEY

1 Start with about 1 tablespoon of fresh herbs (1½ teaspoons of dried herbs) to every 2 cups of mild honey in these proportions and adjust the quantity of herbs to your taste. Bruise the herbs and tie them up in a cheesecloth sack.

2 Heat releases the flavor into the honey. Pour the honey into a stainless steel or glass saucepan and add the sack of herbs, stirring so honey covers it. Heat until the honey is just warm.

3 Pour the honey, and the sack of herbs, into a glass canning jar, tighten the lid, and let the honey rest in a dark cupboard at room temperature for a week. Pour the honey back into the saucepan and reheat until it is just warm. Remove the sack of herbs, pressing down on it with a wooden spoon to extract as much flavor as possible, and pour the honey into hot, sterilized jars. Refrigerate or, if you want to keep the honey on a shelf or give it for gifts, seal the jars.

As a variation, you can mince your herbs very finely and add them directly to the honey instead of tying them in cheesecloth. You can leave the little flecks of herbs in to give the honey a lovely "herbal" appearance, or you can strain them out before the final bottling if you prefer.

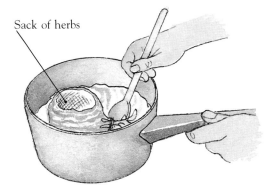

Sack of herbs

▲ **Herbal honey** *smells so good that you'll have a hard time resisting a few tastes while you stir.*

Basic Herbal Jelly

Use mint, parsley, rosemary, sage, tarragon, or thyme as the basis for the infusion in this recipe.

Infusion

2½ cups water

4 Tbsp. dried herbs OR
10 Tbsp. fresh herbs

Boil the water and then pour over the herbs. Let stand 15 minutes. Strain and place in a stainless steel or glass saucepan.

Jelly

¼ cup cider vinegar
2½ cups honey

2 cups strong infusion
3 oz. fruit pectin

Add vinegar and honey to the pan holding the infusion. Bring to a boil, stirring constantly. Add the pectin and, still stirring, boil the mixture for 1 minute. Remove from heat, skim off any foam, and pour into four or five sterilized jelly jars. Seal.

Jellies are some of the prettiest products you'll ever make from your herb garden.

Rose Geranium Jelly

2½ cups mild honey
¾ cup water
16 rose geranium leaves

3 oz. fruit pectin
2 Tbsp. lemon juice
4 sterilized jelly jars

Combine honey, water, and 12 leaves in a stainless steel or glass saucepan. Bring to a boil and add pectin, stirring constantly. Bring to full boil. Add lemon juice, and remove from heat. Remove leaves. Place a fresh leaf in each jar and pour in jelly. Seal; store for at least a month before serving.

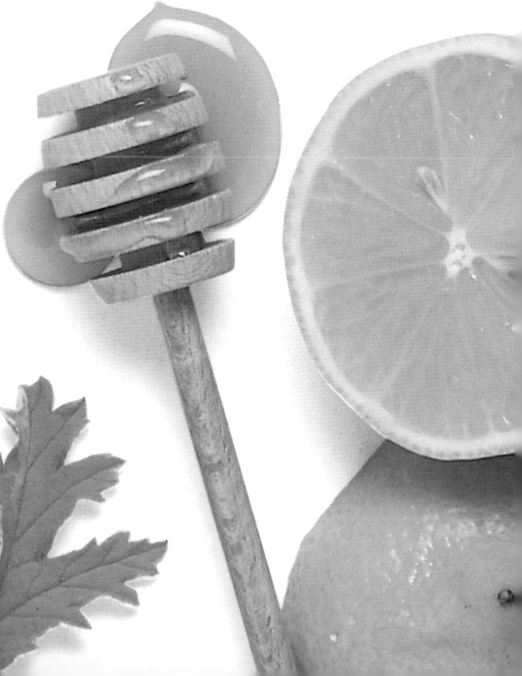

Herbal Breads

Breads and herbs go together as well as bread and butter. But herbs are much healthier for you than butter. When you begin using more herbs in your baking, you'll discover how drastically they reduce the need for butter, cheese, and even sugar.

You can slip herbs into any bread, roll, biscuit, or cracker you make. The only trick is to coordinate the herbal flavoring with whatever else you are serving with the bread. Use the same herbs you would use to flavor the main course. Biscuits made to go with a turkey dinner are delicious flavored with parsley, sage, rosemary, and thyme, for example.

Both fresh and dried herbs work well in baked goods. How much to use depends on your personal taste, of course, but in general, about 1 teaspoon of a fresh, strongly flavored herb such as tarragon or dill will flavor one loaf of bread or a dozen biscuits. Use larger quantities of milder-flavored herbs such as parsley, chervil, and lovage, beginning by adding 2 teaspoons the first time you make the bread and then adjusting amounts to your taste. If you use dried herbs instead of fresh, cut these amounts in half or you may overpower the bread.

If making bread simply doesn't fit into your schedule, you can add herbs to store-bought dough for bread, rolls, or pizza. It takes only a moment to flatten out a thawed loaf of bread dough, sprinkle some fresh or dried herbs over it, and roll it up into a loaf shape again. For preformed rolls, make a depression with your thumb to sprinkle in the herbs. Pizza dough gives you incredible scope, since you only need to press the herbs into the top of it, brush olive oil over them, and then add your toppings. Complement the flavors of a Greek pizza by dusting the dough with 1 teaspoon of fresh thyme, 2 teaspoons of fresh oregano, and 2 tablespoons of fresh Italian parsley before you top it with feta cheese, tomatoes, olives, and onions. If you're making vegetarian or chicken pizzas, liven up the flavors by sprinkling the pizza dough with 2 or 3 teaspoons of one of the lemon herbs – lemon balm, lemon mint, lemon thyme, or lemon verbena – along with freshly ground black pepper, before you add the toppings.

Your herb garden can also add a new dimension to any sweet breads or cakes you make. Anise, lemon verbena, and lemon balm make the flavors more complex. Angelica and sweet cicely allow you to cut from a quarter to an eighth of the sweetener you usually use in the recipe. Whatever you're baking, let your imagination roam through the herb garden to pick the perfect accompaniment.

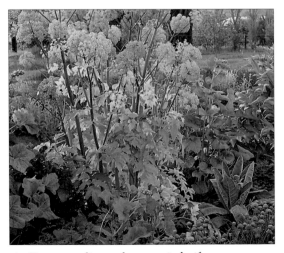

▲ **Grow** *angelica and sweet cicely if you want to cut down on the sugar in your baking – both add a sweet flavor.*

MAKING HERBAL BREAD

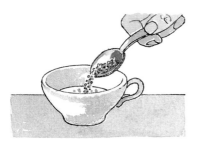

1 *Begin your herbal bread by adding 1 Tbsp. of yeast to ½ cup of warm water. Let stand for 5 to 10 minutes.*

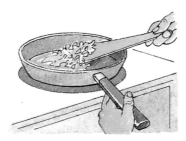

2 *Sauté 2 Tbsp. of chopped onions. Separately, bring 1½ cups of milk to the scalding point. Pour milk into a bowl.*

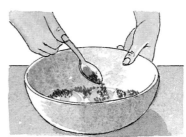

3 *To the milk, add yeast mixture, 4 Tbsp. of oil, 1 Tbsp. of honey, 1 tsp. of salt and 2 eggs. Stir in 5 cups of unbleached white flour to form dough.*

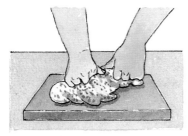

4 *Before kneading, add sautéed onions, 1 Tbsp. of sage, 3 Tbsp. of parsley, 2 tsp. of thyme, and 1 tsp. of rosemary, all chopped finely.*

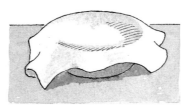

5 *Knead the dough until it is smooth. Place it in an oiled bowl, cover, and let rise.*

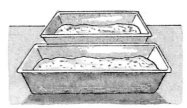

6 *Punch down the dough after 1 hour and form into 2 loaves. Let rise for 45 minutes.*

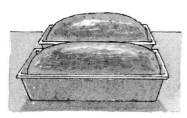

7 *Bake the bread at 400°F for roughly 1 hour or until loaves sound hollow when tapped.*

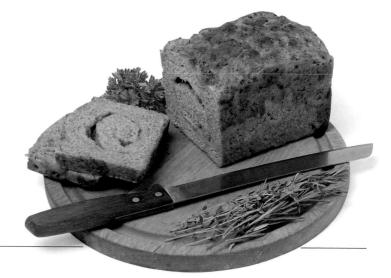

Chapter

4

HERBS FOR HEALTH AND BEAUTY

THE PLEASURES OF HERBS *don't stop when you leave the kitchen. Whether you're seeking a soul-satisfying scent to add to your bath, a little something to help you get to sleep, or a safe and pleasant-smelling way to repel pests from your home, look no further than your herb garden. In this chapter, you'll learn how to make some simple, but effective, home remedies to help cure what ails you. In addition, discover how to make your own customized herbal hair and skin care products, as well as aromatic herb blends for your bath. Brighten your table with fresh arrangements of herb flowers and foliage, or turn dried herbs into sweet-smelling wreaths, swags, and potpourris. Finally, don't forget the family pets. A small patch of catnip is just the thing to keep Fluffy purring, and Fido will wag his tail over a cushion stuffed with flea-repelling herbs.*

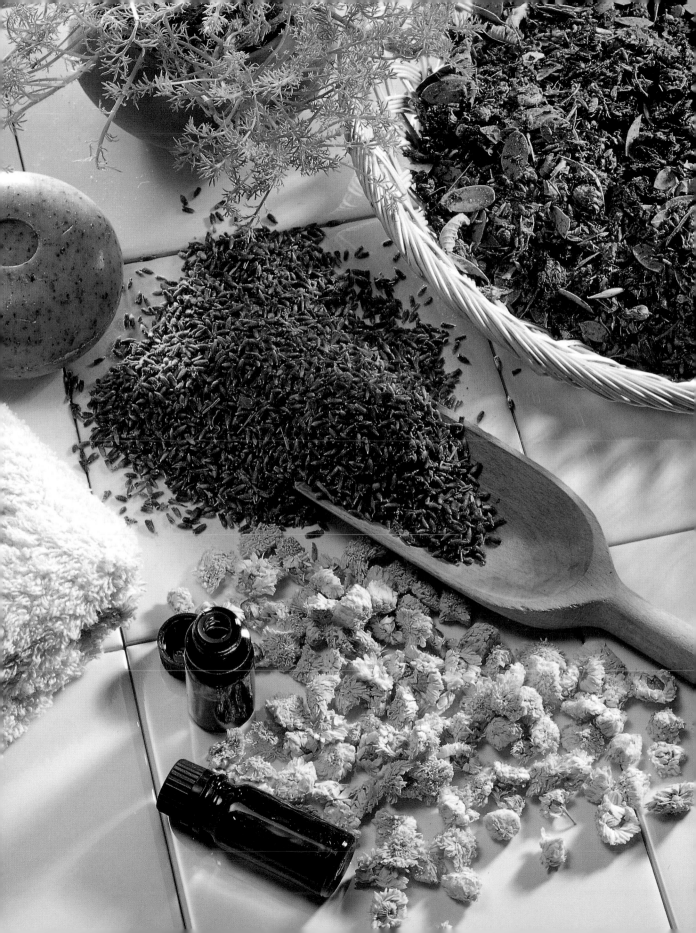

Herbs and Your Health

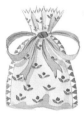

Herbs were the first medicines. Down through the ages, people discovered the medicinal qualities of the plants that grew around them. Today, pharmaceutical companies still use many of these herbs (or synthesized versions of them) in both over-the-counter and prescription medications.

Homemade herbal remedies were once the mainstay of a family's medical care. Although today we depend on commercial medicines, herbal remedies may still soothe a cough or ease a headache as well as any over-the-counter cure. But using herbs medicinally requires caution. The strong active ingredients in some herbs can be dangerous if you use them inappropriately. It's also hard to gauge the strength of an herb; the medicinal qualities can vary depending on how much rain or sun there's been, or other vagaries of cultivation.

Whenever you are using an herb medicinally, be cautious rather than carefree. Be sure your urge to experiment is matched by a healthy dose of common sense. Don't use the remedies in old herbals; according to modern research, many of them are questionable or even harmful. Some of

the herbs in the old recipes have been shown to be carcinogenic in large doses and others seem to be ineffectual. If you want to try a home remedy, be sure to consult a modern herbal. Follow the directions for making and using the remedy to the very letter. There's no need to repeat the "errors" of the trial-and-error learning that helped build our herbal knowledge.

Many people use herb teas medicinally with no ill effects. Chamomile tea is a recommended sleep aid, and a cup of peppermint tea helps to soothe an upset stomach. Healing salves often feature herbs such as aloe. Your herbal home remedies are unlikely to replace your family doctor, but herbs can play a useful role in your medicine cabinet as well as in the kitchen.

BREWING A STRONG DOSE: MAKING INFUSIONS

Infusions are the most commonly used home remedy. They're simply very strong teas that capture the volatile oils in various herbs. To make an infusion, you steep the herbs for at least 20 minutes in a tightly stoppered container. How often you take an infusion depends on its intended result. If you're taking an infusion meant to promote sleep, you take it only once, about 15 minutes before you retire. Infusions for headaches or muscle tension are taken two or three times a day, between meals. Label and refrigerate any infusions that you don't use immediately. Even under refrigeration, they keep for only three days, so make no more than a three-day supply at one time.

CRUSHED AND SIMMERED HERBS: MAKING DECOCTIONS

Decoctions are made by first crushing the herbs to release compounds bound up in the plant tissue, then gently simmering the herbs in water.

MEASURING INGREDIENTS

Calculating the amount of herbs you'll need for medicinal recipes requires different ways of measuring, depending on what you're making.

When making infusions and decoctions:
1 tsp. dried herb = 1 Tbsp. (3 tsp.) fresh herb

When making tinctures:
1 tsp. dried herb = 2 tsp. fresh herb

Typically made from roots, decoctions tend to be stronger than infusions. Decoctions will keep for three days, under refrigeration.

Always pay close attention to the directions for making decoctions; they will vary depending on the herbs used. Many recipes, for example, call for simmering the herbs until the amount of water in the pan is reduced by half, in order to concentrate the medicinal ingredients. This works well with comfrey, but it isn't a good idea with valerian root, which would lose valuable volatile oils to evaporation during simmering. In the case of valerian, the recipe will tell you to tightly cover the simmering pot to capture the oils that might otherwise evaporate.

Be sure you understand the recommended uses of your various decoctions. Comfrey root, for example, makes a wonderful skin salve. However, it is one of the herbs that contemporary research shows to be carcinogenic if ingested in large quantities, so save it for external use only.

SOOTHING AND SOFTENING YOUR SKIN: MAKING SALVES AND OILS

You can use herbal salves both medicinally and cosmetically. Salves are made by combining an herbal decoction with vegetable oil, beeswax, and either gum benzoin or tincture of benzoin. The gum benzoin or tincture of benzoin in the salve helps to preserve it so you can keep it in a labeled, covered jar, stored in a cool, dark location, for many months.

Some herbs, such as lavender and calendula, are used interchangeably. Lavender salve relieves the symptoms of eczema, softens skin as it is healing from burns, and clears bronchial tubes if you apply it just under your nose when you have a cold. But you don't have to restrict your use of this salve to medicinal needs. It also makes a wonderful daily hand cream or body lotion. Calendula blossom salve softens skin, too, and is an effective "post-gardening" treatment for your hands. Comfrey salve is even more curative. If your hands have been roughened and dried by a

MAKING A SALVE

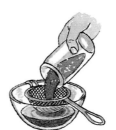

1 *Make comfrey salve by first making and straining 1 cup of a strong decoction.*

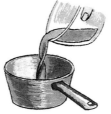

2 *Put 1¼ cups of cold-pressed vegetable oil in a saucepan and add decoction.*

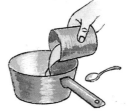

3 *Boil gently until the water evaporates and the oil stops bubbling.*

4 *Slowly melt 1⅛ oz. of beeswax in a small juice can in a pan of water.*

5 *Pour beeswax into the oil, add ¼ tsp. of gum or tincture of benzoin, and stir.*

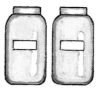

6 *Pour the salve into clean jars, label, and store in cool dark place.*

session of tree pruning in cold, raw weather, for example, apply a liberal dose of comfrey salve to promote fast healing.

MAKING HERBAL OILS

You can also keep your skin soft and supple with herbal oils made from any of the herbs used in salves. Oils are lighter than salves, and you may find you prefer them for daily use. Here's how to make an herbal skin oil using lavender or calendula:

1 Fill a clear glass jar with fresh lavender leaves and flowers or with fresh calendula petals.

2 Crush the herbs with the end of a wooden spoon.

3 Pour in virgin olive oil to cover.

4 Cap the jar and place it on a sunny windowsill. Every other day or so, shake it up to mix in the volatile oils that are being released.

5 After several weeks, strain the oil through thin cotton fabric. Press the herbs against the fabric with your fingers to release all of the herb's essential oils.

6 Pour the oil into glass jars, label, and store in a dark, dry place. It will keep for up to a year.

POWERFUL SMALL DOSES:
MAKING TINCTURES

Tinctures are concentrated doses of herbal remedies. Of the herbs listed in the Directory, only betony and feverfew are used in tinctures. Betony tincture is used to treat tension headaches, while feverfew is believed to help relieve migraines.

Because of their strength, you use tinctures in very small dosages – squeezing 10 to 15 drops from a glass medicine dropper just under your tongue. One dose is often all that's needed; if not, wait several hours before taking a second. Do not exceed four doses a day.

Store tinctures in labeled dark-colored jars. They'll keep for as long as a year.

MAKING A TINCTURE

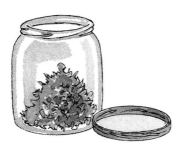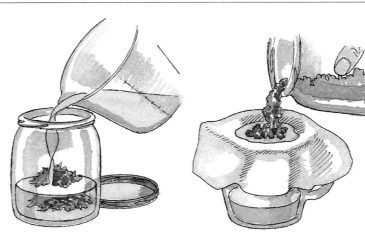

1 *Make a tincture by placing 4 oz. of dried betony in a jar with a tight-fitting plastic lid.*

2 *Add 2½ cups of alcohol to the herbs. Most people use brandy or vodka.*

3 *Shake every day for two weeks, then strain out the herbs. Label, and store in a dark place.*

ABOUT AROMATHERAPY

Aromatherapy is the increasingly popular practice of using scents as part of a therapeutic regime. Based on the idea that certain fragrances have particular effects on the mind and body, most aromatherapy depends on essential oils. These oils are added to massage oils or toiletries, applied as perfumes, added to bathwater or steaming water, applied to hot or cold compresses, or simply inhaled.

You can use your homegrown herbs in aromatherapy preparations. Simply use one of the herbs below, or a combination of them, in the recipes for oils, potpourris, cosmetics, and other fragrant concoctions you'll find throughout this chapter.

Many store-bought aromatherapy products use essential oils. But few of us have either the equipment to distill our own oils or the enormous quantities of herbs required. For example, it takes 600 pounds of roses to produce 1 ounce of essential oil! However, it's easy to make your own delightfully fragrant oil extract by infusing unscented oils like safflower oil with your homegrown herbs. You can use your homemade oils to add aroma to your bath or to apply to your skin. When stronger concentrations are needed, commercially made essential oils are a practical alternative to making your own – only a few drops are needed to produce the desired fragrant effect.

Oil	Uses	Properties	Oil	Uses	Properties
Bee balm (Bergamot)	Essential oil used in perfumes and as an inhalant. Leaves and flowers used in bathwater, potpourris.	Antidepressant.	Lavender	Essential oil used in perfumes, toiletries. Leaves and flowers used in bathwater, potpourris, compresses.	Calming, purifying. Improves mental clarity, relieves tension headaches and insomnia. The oil is a disinfectant.
Chamomile	Essential oil used as an inhalant. Flowers used in bathwater, steaming water.	Calming. Diminishes anger.	Peppermint	Use leaves in bathwater or add to steaming water on the stove.	Brightens moods, energizes. Improves mental clarity and memory.
Cilantro	Essential oil used as an inhalant or in bathwater. Crushed seeds (coriander) used in bathwater, steaming water.	Stimulating, energizing.	Rosemary	Essential oil is added to massage oils and baths. Leaves used in baths, steaming water, compresses.	Energizes, relaxes tense muscles, brightens moods, increases mental clarity. The oil is a disinfectant.
Geraniums, scented	Essential oil of rose-scented geranium used in perfumes, potpourris, toiletries, bathwater, steaming water. Leaves are added to potpourris, bathwater, steaming water. Other scented geraniums may be used in bathwater, potpourris, steaming water.	Rose geranium is calming, restores emotional balance and peacefulness. Sharp-scented geraniums are energizing; sweet-scented types are calming.			

Herbs for Beauty

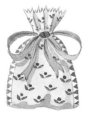

From scented baths to skin splashes, hair rinses to eyewashes, herbal toiletries let you indulge yourself with pleasure. Best of all, most of them are as easy to make as a simple infusion.

Herbal baths are wonderfully relaxing. You can use a single herb, such as lavender, or a mixture of herbs like lemon verbena, mint, and rosemary. Fill a muslin sack with the herb leaves of your choice and hang it just under the faucet so the water flows over it as it fills the tub, or add a strong infusion of herbs to your bathwater for a gentle scent.

Use your herbs to treat yourself to a pleasing array of homemade herbal skin care products. They're marvelously effective and make delightful gifts for yourself or your friends. By combining your herbs with different ingredients, you can create customized cosmetics for dry or oily skin. The lavender oil recipe in "Making Herbal Oils" on page 84, for example, is an excellent moisturizer for dry skin. If you have oily skin, make a lavender astringent instead. Follow the same procedure described for the oil, but substitute good-quality white wine vinegar for the olive oil. To get the full benefit of lavender's aromatic and antiseptic qualities, repeat the process three times, adding a fresh supply of herbs to the same vinegar each time. The resulting product is more effective and more pleasing to the nose than most commercial astringents.

THE MAKINGS OF A MASK

Create a refreshing face mask with herbs from your own garden. Here are suggested herbs to use and instructions for mixing up your own herbal facial.

For normal skin, use fennel or mint. For dry skin, choose comfrey. For oily skin, try either sage or yarrow. To exfoliate dead skin and refine pores, use 2 tablespoons of pounded fennel seed.

1   Add 1 cup of fresh herbs (or 3 tablespoons of dried herbs, soaked overnight in a small amount of distilled water) to 2 tablespoons of distilled water and 2 tablespoons of organic oatmeal.
2   Mix in a blender or food processor.
3   Apply the resulting mixture and leave it on your skin for at least 15 minutes before rinsing. Apply your herbal mask in the evening, before bed, since it can cause your skin to flush.

You can also make a great astringent with mint:

1 Finely chop 4 tablespoons of mint. Add the chopped mint to 4 tablespoons of cider vinegar.

2 Let the mixture infuse on a sunny windowsill for about a week; shake it daily.

3 Strain out the chopped mint. Add 2½ cups of distilled water.

4 Pour the mixture into dark-colored glass bottles and label. Shake before using.

You can make massage oils the same way you make lavender oil – with one important exception. Instead of olive oil, use a lighter oil like almond, avocado, or safflower.

BEAUTIFUL HAIR THE HERBAL WAY

Herbs work wonders for your hair. Using your own herbs, you can make shampoos and rinses that give your hair bounce and shine.

Herbal hair rinses can help you wash away excess oiliness. To make a rinse for oily hair, use any of the herbs listed under "to condition oily hair" in "Herbs for Hair Care" on this page. To make a rinse, finely chop 1 cup of fresh herbs and add them to a pan filled with 1 quart of distilled or soft water. Bring the water to a simmer; simmer for 15 minutes. Remove the pot from the stove, cover, and let it infuse for about an hour. Strain the infusion and stir in 1 quart of cider vinegar. Pour into plastic bottles, label, and store in a dark, cool place. Use about a cup of the rinse after shampooing your hair.

Try some herbal conditioners too. There's no need to rinse out these fragrant solutions. Choose the herbs that provide the conditioning effect you want from "Herbs for Hair Care." Mince 1 cup of herbs, add to 2 cups of distilled or soft water, and simmer for 15 minutes. Let the infusion steep for an hour, and then add 1 tablespoon of glycerin, one drop at a time, while stirring vigorously. Pour into a plastic bottle, label, and store in a cool, dark place. To use, comb about ½ teaspoon of conditioner into your hair while it's wet.

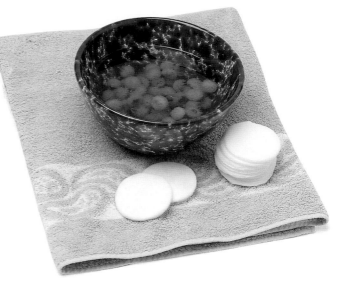

▲ **Pure luxury** – *there's no other way to describe having a good supply of homemade beauty-care products.*

HERBS FOR HAIR CARE

Herbal shampoos can make your hair look better than ever. To create your own custom blend, make a strong decoction of the herb of your choice from the list below, and add 2 tablespoons of the decoction to a normal application of mild baby shampoo.

- **To condition dry hair:** comfrey, parsley, or sage
- **To condition oily hair:** calendula, lavender, lemon balm, mint, rosemary, southernwood, or yarrow
- **To prevent dandruff:** chamomile, parsley, rosemary, southernwood, or thyme
- **To give your hair body:** calendula, nasturtium, parsley, rosemary, sage, or southernwood
- **To soothe scalp irritation:** catnip, chamomile, or comfrey

Custom-Blend Potpourri

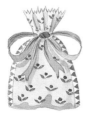

A real potpourri, made with herbs from your own garden and high-quality essential oils and fixatives, is completely different from the sickly sweet mixtures you can buy in stores. All-natural ingredients are more pleasing than the too-sweet synthetics.

You can blend a potpourri fragrance to suit the environment where you'll use it – making a spicy scent for the kitchen, a calming lemony combination for the bedroom, or a bracing minty mixture for the family room. Natural potpourris are also much more beautiful to look at than the commercial mixes, which use wood shavings and dyed plant materials.

MATCH THE MOOD

The best potpourris are complex blends of various fragrances. Use "About Aromatherapy" on page 85 to help you decide which fragrances you want to stand out in various potpourris. For example, in the bathroom you might want the clean smell of lavender. Rose might be more appropriate for a bedroom, while a spicy mixture of sweet marjoram, vanilla bean, mint, and cinnamon is wonderful in a kitchen.

Most of the scented material in a potpourri will come from your herb garden. But don't hesitate to buy other perfumed ingredients, such as dried roses, cinnamon sticks, Greek myrtle leaves, or bayberries. You can find interesting materials at the grocery store or a well-stocked natural food store. Less common ingredients, such as bayberries and Greek myrtle leaves, are available through specialty mail-order suppliers

like those listed in "Resources" on page 155.

The other key ingredients in a potpourri are essential oils and a fixative. Essential oils of rose, lavender, bergamot, and other delicious fragrances add concentrated, long-lasting scent to your mixture. Fixatives, such as orrisroot and oakmoss, keep the fragrance of your potpourri strong and fresh for a long time, just as their name suggests.

VISUAL APPEAL

Potpourris are often kept in a bowl or dish, where their naturally decorative look is as much an asset as their delectable fragrance. You may want to include other dried materials, even if they aren't fragrant, to pep up your potpourri with color. From your flower garden, add blossoms that hold

---

A CALMING MIXTURE

Make a potpourri with a wonderful soothing scent by mixing these ingredients in a plastic tub with a tight-fitting lid:

2 cups lavender florets
2 cups lemon verbena leaves
2 cups mint leaves
1½ cups calendula flower petals
1 cup chamomile flowers
1 cup lemon-scented geranium leaves
½ cup rosemary leaves
1 oz. shredded angelica root
4 oz. orrisroot

Add 10 drops of oil of lavender to the herbal mix. Tape the lid closed with duct tape. Shake the closed container to thoroughly mix all ingredients and then store it in a dark, warm place for six weeks. Shake the container daily. Pour the potpourri into a decorative bowl when finished.

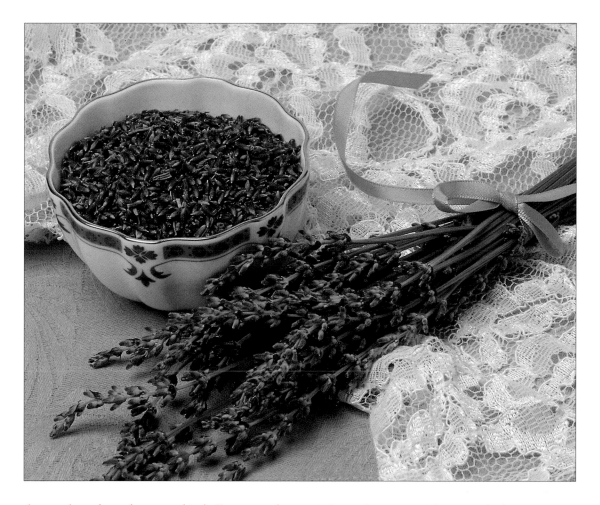

their color when they are dried. For example, dried delphinium florets are a lovely blue color that seems well suited to lavender-scented potpourris.

Dried annual or perennial statice, strawflowers, or gomphrena are other good choices for a bit of color. Break the statice into florets and pull individual petals from strawflowers or gomphrena and add them to the potpourri just before you mix in the essential oil.

HOW TO MAKE A MIX

Make your first potpourris by following a recipe, like the one in "A Calming Mixture" opposite. Then have fun experimenting with your own combinations and proportions.

▲ **Lavender** *is one of the easiest herbs to grow and use in potpourri mixtures. Just a few plants will supply all you'll need.*

Follow these basic guidelines to create a pleasing mix:

1 Include six to eight different ingredients in a potpourri mix, using roughly 1 to 2 cups of each ingredient. If you want to make a potpourri with fewer ingredients, simply maintain the proportions of fixative and essential oils to quantity of plant material described in Step 2.

2 For every 6 to 10 cups of potpourri material, add 4 to 8 tablespoons of a fixative material and 10 to 20 drops of an essential oil.

Pillows and Sachets

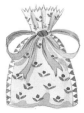

Herbal pillows and sachets are a treat to have around the house, and they make delightful gifts. It takes only a couple of hours to make these fragrant offerings.

Try your hand at sweet-scented sachets for dresser drawers or the linen closet. Or keep your teapot nice and warm with a woodsy or spicy tea cozy and a set of matching mug coasters. You can easily fashion herbal inserts, filled with calming and sleep-promoting scents, for your bed pillows. Or use the power of herbs to create flea-repellent cushions (see page 97) for your pets.

PILLOW FILLINGS

Make the filling for an herbal pillow just as you would make a potpourri mixture. Use a light hand with sweet, floral scents. Woodsy and spicy fragrances are refreshing in herbal pillows. A potpourri scented with pine needles adds a subtle character to a room, while a mixture that's heavy with lavender may be fine in a potpourri, but cloying in a larger pillow. Think about how you want to use your herbal accents. If you use a strong floral mix inside a coaster pad or tea cozy, for instance, it will interfere with the aroma of the tea you are drinking. Instead, enhance the flavor by filling your coasters with a potpourri made from the herbs you generally use for tea – mints, lemon balm, catnip, and chamomile.

Whether or not you use essential oils and fixatives depends on how you'll be using the finished pillow. You won't need essential oils for sleep pillows, moth repellents, and pet cushions – for these items, the fresh, natural herbal scents are enough. Include fixatives, such as oakmoss or gum benzoin, in everything but insect-repellent mixtures. You'll want a fine-textured stuffing mixture so that the herbs' stems and leaves don't make bulges in the pillow. An easy way to get the right texture is to pour a finished potpourri into a wide-mesh strainer held over a large bowl. Shake the strainer to sift out the small pieces. You can pop this fine material right into a pillow casing and tuck it into a drawer or linen closet.

All potpourris eventually lose their fragrance. To revive the scent, crush the herbs in the pillow between your fingers. Eventually, after three to six months, your herbs will lose most of their scent. Simply open up the pillow, compost the old potpourri, and fill with a fresh batch.

PILLOWCASES FOR YOUR HERBS

Choose tightly woven fabric for your pillows to keep the stuffing mixture where it belongs. If your herbal pillows will be moved and handled, sew the edges shut, using a fine stitch.

If you're placing a sachet in a drawer or closet,

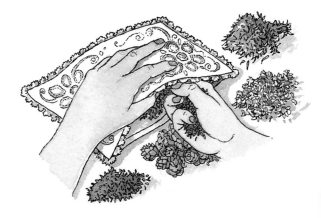

▲ **Dream pillows** *contain catnip, hyssop, chamomile, lavender, and sometimes hops.*

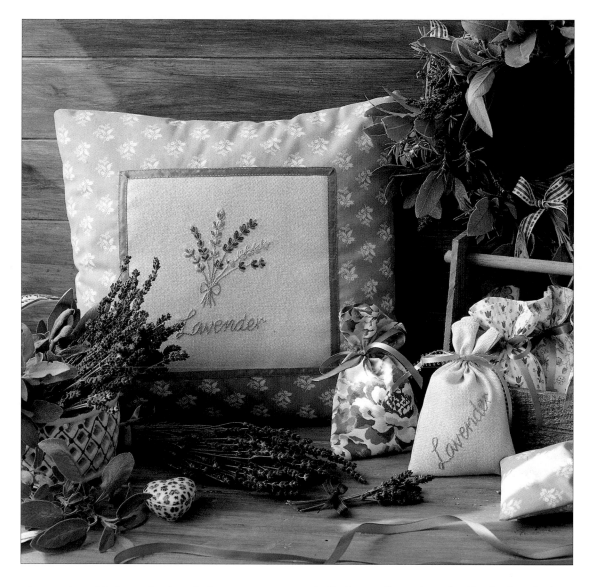

where it's unlikely to be handled, cut a 4- to 6-inch-square of fabric, fill it with your herb mixture, and pull up the corners to make a bundle. Tie the bundle with a rubber band and then add a decorative ribbon. Leave a loop from the ribbon to hang the pillow from a clothes rod or closet hook. Every time you open the closet door, you'll be greeted by a lovely fragrance. Your clothes will pick up just a hint of it, too, although it won't be strong enough to interfere with any perfume or cologne you might choose to wear.

▲ **Sachets,** *pillows, lavender "bottles," and other fragrant garden creations become treasures for the home and wonderful gifts. Make a collection of pillow and sachet covers from pretty fabric scraps and fill them with a variety of homemade potpourris.*

Herb Bouquets

A fresh herbal bouquet can be as beautiful as anything you'll find at the florist shop. Rich textures and subtle colors make a bouquet of herbs a pleasure to see as well as sniff. Combine the blue-purple spikes of anise hyssop with the cheerful yellow and orange faces of calendulas, and you have a simple arrangement fit for company dinner. Or fill a jelly jar with sprigs of ruffled purple basil and golden-leaved thyme for a kitchen-counter accent.

▶ **A fresh bouquet** of herbs is every bit as colorful and fragrant as a more traditional floral arrangement.

If you can't spare enough herbs to make a generous bouquet all by themselves, use a few stems of beautiful herb foliage to accent bouquets of garden flowers. Contrast a bunch of vivid red zinnias with light green lemon balm leaves, or use trailing pieces of thyme to balance an upright cluster of clove-scented pinks.

DESIGNING FOR EYE APPEAL

Start your herbal bouquet with a "foundation plant" that supplies the dominant design element. Using one main plant as the focus of your arrangement makes more of a statement than a lot of different plants, just as a group of the same plants in the garden packs a bigger punch than a mixed, one-here, one-there planting. Add pizzazz to your design with colorful flowers or foliage. Repeat the same colors throughout the bouquet or place vivid colors at strategic points in it.

For example, you might want to create a large bouquet for a table in your entrance hallway. Since the arrangement is to be large, you'll need a tall plant for the foundation. Red bee balm, borage, southernwood, or wormwood are good

choices. Set the foundation plants into a floral "rose" or a piece of floral foam in the bottom of a vase, and cut and arrange until they please your eye. Now comes the fun – begin filling in the basic design with the highlights. Use pretty leaves and flower spikes that you've selected for their colors or their interesting textures or branching shapes. Snip and place, place, snip, and place again until the design is an herbal work of art waiting to greet you at the door.

Smaller herbal bouquets are just as charming and easy to put together on the spur of the moment. On a dinner table, for instance, a simple rounded bouquet of violets or nasturtiums is a natural. Or you can get more imaginative with your designs: Start by putting a bunch of parsley in a round vase, leaving just enough space around the stems so you can slip in additional herbs. If it's spring, add violets and short sprigs of variegated sage, rue, and lemon thyme to the bowl. In summer, try a combination of hyssop blooms, purple basil, and chive blossoms, interspersing them among the ferny green parsley for a purple-hued arrangement. Or make a cheery bunch of parsley mixed with feverfew, garlic chive flowers (these smell like roses, not garlic), and calendula.

HIDDEN MESSAGES

From medieval to Victorian times, herbs and flowers were used to convey messages between friends (and sometimes between enemies!). Today, so few people remember the "language of herbs" that it helps to include a translation. Choose a bouquet according to what you want to tell the recipient. Don't forget to include a note explaining the message.

Herb	Meaning	Herb	Meaning
Aloe	Healing, protection	Marjoram, sweet	Joy, happiness
Angelica	Inspiration	Mint	Wisdom
Basil, sweet	Best wishes, friendship	Nasturtium	Conquest
Bee balm	Virtue	Parsley	Celebration, festivity
Borage	Courage, bravery	Rosemary	Remembrance
Calendula	Sadness, hopelessness	Rue	Repentance, grief
Chamomile	Wisdom, patience, resignation	Saffron	Marriage
		Sage	Wisdom, long life
Chervil	Sincerity	Santolina	Virtue
Chives	Usefulness	Savory	Interest
Cilantro	Hidden worth, hidden feelings	Southernwood	Constancy
Dill	Good cheer, fortitude in adversity	Sweet woodruff	Humility
		Tansy	Hostility
Fennel	Strength, endurance	Tarragon, French	Lasting involvement
Geranium, scented	Happiness	Thyme	Daring
Hyssop	Cleanliness	Valerian	Conciliation
Lavender	Silence, recognition and acceptance of love	Violet	Modesty
Lemon balm	Sympathy, regeneration	Yarrow	Good health

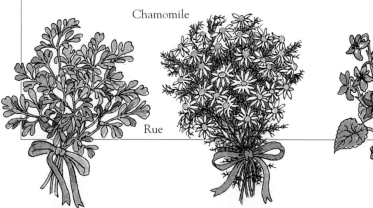

Chamomile

Rue

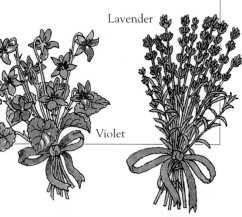

Lavender

Violet

Dried Arrangements

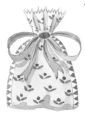

Winter is an ideal time to make dried arrangements, but planning for this pleasure really begins the year before. You need a lot of dried herbs to make beautiful full wreaths and generous arching swags.

Think ahead when you make out your spring seed order and draw your garden designs. You'll want to grow plenty of the herbs that dry well – anise hyssop, bee balm, tansy, wormwood, and yarrow. For variety's sake, plant several different colors of bee balm and as many different yarrows as you can fit into the garden. If space is limited, choose 'Summer Pastels' yarrow, a mixture that includes many different colors.

When you gather herbs for future use in winter bouquets, cut the stems as long as possible. Hang the herbs as described in "Hanging to Dry" on page 62, allowing plenty of room around them so that air can circulate freely. Then pack them away until the day when making winter bouquets seems like the perfect thing to do.

CREATING INSPIRED ARRANGEMENTS

A vase filled with a burst of golden tansy or yarrow is simplicity itself, and it's so bright and cheerful it can add light to any room. It's hard to stick with simple arrangements, though, once you have a wealth of dried herbs. Add purple hyssop flowers or lavender chive blossoms to your simple yellow bouquet and you have a whole different look. From there, it's just a short trip to the drying room to look for bee balm flowers, silvery santolina, and all kinds of other delights.

In the summertime, forage in your yard for wild grasses and other interesting weeds, as well as seedpods from milkweed and other "weedy" plants, for use in fall and winter arrangements. Look for berries, too, and put aside a few woody branches, with or without berries, to add backbone to your dried bouquets.

Just as with fresh arrangements, you'll want to start your dried bouquets by choosing a basic foundation plant. Then weave in colors and foliage accents to create a pleasing shape. Imagination is the key to having a good time and

▼ **Combine** *dried herbs, flowers, and foliage to create a wreath that's bursting with color and fragrance. Here, roses, lavender, chive flowers, feverfew, and lady's mantle brighten a base of sage and lamb's-ears.*

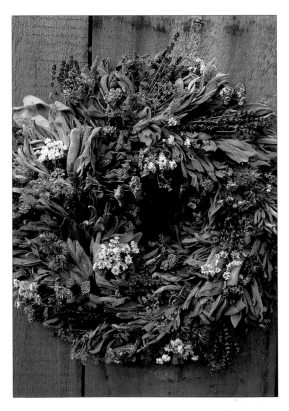

▶ **Adorn** *your rafters with bunches of drying herbs for an effect that's both pleasant and practical. You can enjoy the beauty of the herbs as they dry and have materials for wreaths and arrangements close at hand.*

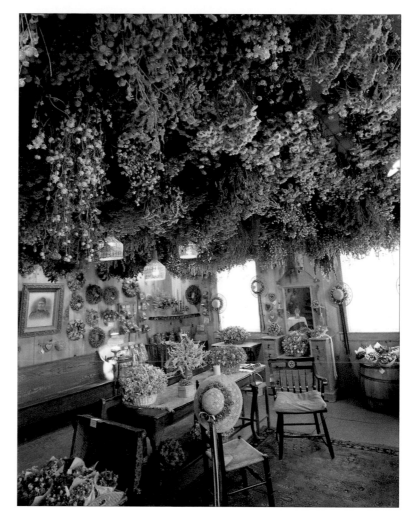

making designs that you'll be pleased to display. Save all the materials that are too small or too large for your bouquet, to use in other creations. Pieces with small stems are perfect for tucking into a wreath or brightening potpourri; those that branch too widely make a good base for a door arrangement.

STORING DRIED MATERIALS

If you dry large quantities of herbs for winter bouquets, you'll probably need to store them for a few weeks to several months before you're ready to use them.

To keep them in the best condition, protect them from both light and high humidity. You'll also want to keep insects and rodents away from any seedpods that may seem like a nice winter pantry for these pests.

Pack the dried materials in large cardboard boxes, lined with plain white tissue paper. Gently set the materials in the box, in a single layer. If they are very lightweight, you can add another layer of tissue paper to the box and fill it with a second layer. Protect it from pests by adding some of the insect-repellent herbs – pennyroyal, santolina, and wormwood. Tape the box shut with duct tape and keep it in a cool, dark, dry area.

Insect Repellents

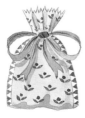

Herbal insect repellents work. They can help keep flies away from the dinner table, fleas off the pets, ants out of the kitchen, moths from eating your woolens, and all but the most hungry mosquitoes away from your skin.

Herbal insect repellents are harmless to people, animals, and the environment. Their clean, fresh scent smells great to our nose, but it's that same sharp fragrance that helps to deter insects. Santolina is particularly effective at repelling insects. It also soothes insect bites and stings. When you're making repellent mixtures, save all the small bits of leaves and flowers that fall off the santolina branches. Crush them into a fine powder and store in a labeled

---

▼ **A pretty bouquet** *of herbs such as rue, peppermint, tansy, and basil adds color to your table and helps keep pesky insects away.*

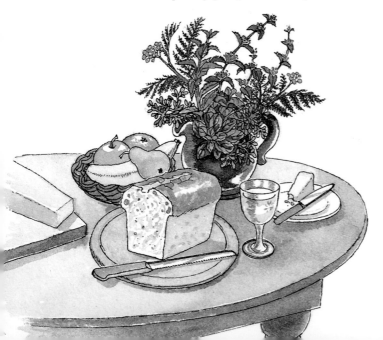

> ### INSECT-REPELLENT SKIN LOTION
> Make an herbal oil, as described in "Making Herbal Oils" on page 84, using pennyroyal, rosemary, and tansy with a light vegetable oil such as soybean or safflower. The strong fragrance of these herbs is the key to deterring insects, so repeat the infusion process three times, using fresh herbs each time to concentrate the aroma. Finish off the lotion by adding at least a teaspoon of purchased essential oil of citronella. Label the lotion and store in a dark, cool location. Rub the lotion on your skin when you venture into insect-infested territory. If any of the ingredients irritate your skin, you can rub a bit on your clothing or onto a bandanna instead. But don't put it on your best clothes – the oil in the lotion will leave a stain.

dark-colored glass jar. The next time someone in your family gets stung by a bee or bitten by a mosquito, rub this powder over the area to help make it feel better.

KEEPING MOTHS AWAY

Moth repellents are an excellent way to introduce yourself to the effectiveness of herbal repellents. Recipes for moth repellents generally include lavender, rosemary, santolina, and southernwood, all of which are offensive to moths. It's fun to make anti-moth sachets, but you can also use these herbs as is by tucking them into tissue paper and laying them among your wool clothes and blankets.

Dry your moth-repelling herbs as usual. Plan to use at least two kinds of anti-moth herbs, and make one of them santolina if possible. When the herbs are completely dry, slip them into an old pillowcase or lay them between sheets of tissue paper. Place the pillowcase or tissue paper in the

Moth-Repellent Sachets

This special potpourri of dried herbs has a pleasant fragrance that moths find repulsive. Package the following lightly scented mixture in squares of cloth as described in "Pillowcases for Your Herbs" on page 90, and hang them in your closet or nestle them amid your sweaters to deter moths.

    6 cups dried santolina leaves
    4 cups dried southernwood leaves
    1 cup dried chamomile leaves
    1 cup dried lavender leaves
    1 cup dried rosemary leaves
    ½ cup crumbled dried bay leaves
    ¼ cup ground cinnamon
    6 oz. orrisroot or oakmoss

Mix the ingredients. Add 20 drops of oil of lavender to the herbal mix. Store in a container, taped shut with duct tape. Shake the closed container to thoroughly mix all ingredients and then store it in a dark, warm place for six weeks. Shake the container daily. Pour the mixture into squares of cloth or pillowcases when finished and place the sachets amid your woolens.

closet or in the boxes or chests where you store woolens. Protect the clothes in your closet by hanging smaller bags of these herbs or a potpourri of them from the clothes rod.

If you store woolens throughout the year, remember to replace the moth-repellent herbs in spring and again in the fall.

Insect repellents for pets

Make your pets' lives more pleasant with herbal insect repellents. These repellents are much safer to use than many of the commercially available solutions because they do not contain poisons. Herb-stuffed cushions in your dog's or cat's bed are an easy and effective way to help keep your pet flea-free. You can also drench pest-troubled pets with a strongly scented herbal dip.

As every cat lover knows, you might as well forget trying to use a dip on most cats. Cats will take to the cushions, though, especially if you add 1 to 1½ cups of catnip to the mixture. You can also soak a cotton collar in the undiluted dip to help repel pests. Buy two collars if you try this and switch them every other day, dipping in the repellent again before you put it on your pet. This collar won't kill fleas like the commercial ones do, but it will diminish the number that move in to raise a family on your pet.

▼ **Fido** *never had it so good – a great place to sleep and no pesky fleas!*

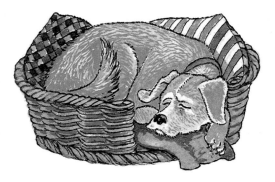

Pet Dip

Limit pest populations on your pet with this refreshing dip. Use it weekly, beginning in early spring.

1 Make a strong infusion by pouring boiling water over 2 to 3 cups each of fresh pennyroyal, peppermint, rosemary, and santolina.

2 Steep the infusion for at least 30 minutes in a covered container.

3 Strain out the herbs and add about a gallon of lukewarm water.

4 Saturate your pet's coat with the mixture. It helps to have a second person to control the pet while you pour the infusion over its body!

Chapter

5

HERB DIRECTORY

❧

Now that you're familiar *with the basic techniques for growing herbs successfully, you're ready to choose the herbs you want to include in your own herb garden. The "Herb Directory" features 51 popular herbs, along with complete information on how to grow, harvest, and use each one.*

For easy reference, you'll find the herbs listed in alphabetical order by common name. Botanical names are included to clear up any confusion that may occur when a plant's common name varies from one region to the next. Each entry is packed with everything you need to know to grow your favorite herbs, using only organic and ecologically sound methods.

HOW TO USE THE HERB DIRECTORY

The sample layout, displayed below, explains the symbols used, as well as all the essential points that are covered for every herb.

Symbols

1 Description

2 How to Grow

5 Cultivars and Relatives

3 Harvesting

4 Uses

6 Tips

UNDERSTANDING THE SYMBOLS

Attention required
Is the plant easy or
demanding to grow?

Easy requiring little
attention

Easy but requires regular
attention

Moderate

Demanding

Friendly to
Does the plant attract
beneficial insects, bees,
and butterflies?

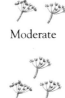 ✓ Yes ✗ No

Ornamental
Is the plant ornamental
as well as useful?

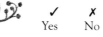 ✓ Yes ✗ No

Container growing
Can the plant be grown
successfully in a
container?

✓ Yes ✗ No

Yield
Does the plant provide a
small, moderate, or
abundant amount of herbs?

 Small

Moderate

Large

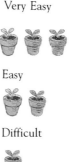 Abundant

Easy to grow
Is the plant easy or
difficult to grow?

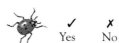 Very Easy

Easy

Difficult

Very difficult

1 Description
Information is given on the life cycle: annual, biennial, or perennial; the plant's height at maturity, the plant's range of hardiness, based on the United States Department of Agriculture Plant Hardiness Zone Map, reproduced on page 154; the appearance of the flowers and leaves; when it blooms; and its flavor and fragrance. This brief description guides you in combining the herb with other plants in a mixed bed, and lets you know what it will look like through the season.

2 How to Grow
This section lets you know how and when to start plants for best results. You'll see what light exposure the plant requires, as well as what its soil fertility and moisture needs are. The spacing information allows you to give just enough but not too much room to each herb. Check this section of the Directory when you're planning your garden, and then again when you're getting plants started.

3 Harvesting
Harvest your herbs when their flavors and fragrances are at their best. Here you'll find which parts of each herb to harvest, when to harvest, and any special techniques to use. You'll also learn the best ways to preserve your herbs for future use.

4 Uses
Discover how versatile your favorite herbs are! This section lists the many ways in which you can use the herbs from your garden. You'll find cooking recommendations for the culinary herbs, as well as medicinal and cosmetic applications, their uses in crafts such as potpourri, and even their suitability as insect repellents.

5 Cultivars and Relatives
Look here to learn about other herbal or ornamental plants that are related to the herb, as well as any particularly excellent cultivars. Occasionally you'll also find warnings about an herb's less-desirable relatives here.

6 Tips
This section gives useful information that is not otherwise covered in the entry. Always read the tips because you'll learn something that can contribute to your gardening success with the particular herb.

Aloe

Aloe barbadensis, formerly A. vera

Aloe is known as the "medicine plant" because the gel inside the leaves is used externally to treat many skin ailments. But even if you never need this plant for its medicinal qualities, you'll appreciate its decorative qualities.

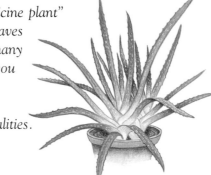

Attention required

  ✗

Friendly to

  ✓

Ornamental

  ✓

Container growing

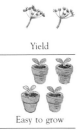

Yield

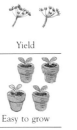

Easy to grow

DESCRIPTION

Perennial
2 to 3 feet tall
Zones 9 and 10; elsewhere as a houseplant
Flowers: Yellow or orange, 1-inch-long tubular flowers borne in a terminal cluster on a 3- to 4-foot-long stalk
Leaves: Fleshy, sword-shaped leaves with spiny edges grow to form a rosette
Flavor and fragrance: Unremarkable; aloe is not commonly used internally.

HOW TO GROW

When to plant: In Zones 9 and 10, plant container-grown plants in the garden anytime. North of Zone 9, grow aloe in a container and overwinter indoors.
Where to plant: Aloe prefers full sun but tolerates partial shade.
Soil and fertility: Plant in well-drained neutral soil (pH 7.0) of average fertility.
Plant spacing: Allow 1 to 2 feet between plants growing outdoors.

Pests: Mealybugs, root mealybugs
Diseases: Susceptible to root rot in consistently moist soil

HARVESTING

When to harvest: Pick leaves anytime during the growing season as needed once they reach a minimum of 5 to 6 inches long.
How to harvest: Cut off the oldest leaves at the base.

USES

Medicinal: This succulent plant is grown in homes around the world for its skin-healing properties. Split the leaf and rub gel from the inside of the leaf over minor burns. Research shows that the gel contains compounds that are anesthetic and antibacterial. If the burn is not too severe, the gel prevents scar tissue from forming and pigmentation returns to normal.

TIPS

Propagate aloe by rooting one of the offshoots that form near the base of the plant. To remove an offshoot, shake the mother plant out of the pot and gently pull the young plantlet away. Use a trowel to separate offshoots from garden-grown plants. The offshoot will already have grown some roots, so you can replant it immediately in a container or, in warm zones, in your garden. Aloe makes a nearly care-free houseplant if it is potted in a fast-draining soil mix and watered only when the top inch of the soil dries out.

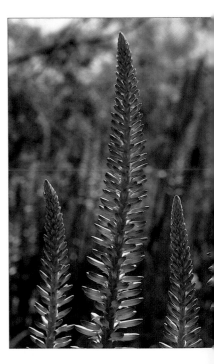

▲ **Aloe** *can be planted in the garden in warm zones. North of Zone 9, it can be planted two weeks after the frost-free date in well-drained soil and full sun.*

Angelica

Angelica archangelica

With leaves that can grow 2 feet long on stems as tall as 8 feet, angelica makes a dramatic focal point for the rear of the herb garden.

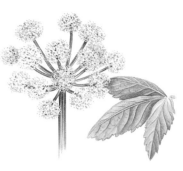

DESCRIPTION

Biennial
5 to 8 feet tall
Zones 4 to 9

Flowers: Great rounded Queen-Anne's-lace-like umbels, up to 10 inches in diameter, consist of many small green honey-scented flowers. Plants bloom in June or July in the second or third year of growth.
Leaves: Broad leaves with toothed edges. Plants die back in winter.
Flavor and fragrance: All plant parts have a mild licorice flavor with a slightly spicy bite. The fragrance is faintly sweet.

HOW TO GROW

When to plant: Angelica seeds must be fresh to germinate. Gather ripe seeds in late summer or early fall and sow where they are to grow – angelica is difficult to transplant. Seeds require light to germinate. Refrigerate purchased seed until planting.
Where to plant: Prefers partial shade but will grow in shade and, if mulched, in sun.

Soil and fertility: Plant in moderately moist, slightly acid soil of average fertility.
Plant spacing: Space plants 2 feet apart.
Pests: Aphids, earwigs, leafminers, spider mites
Diseases: Crown rot

HARVESTING

When to harvest: For best quality, gather leaves and stems in the morning after the dew has dried, in spring and summer but before plants flower. Collect seeds in late summer. Dig roots in early fall after the first year of growth.

How to harvest: Cut stems at a node (where leaf attaches to stem) several inches above ground level. Strip leaves from the cut stems. Enclose whole seed heads when nearly ripe to prevent shattering. Dig roots in dry weather with a spading fork.
Drying: Hang leaves and enclosed seed heads to air dry. Cut roots into 2-inch pieces and dry in a dehydrator.

USES

Cooking: Use seeds in cakes and beverages and chopped stems to sweeten desserts. Cook the leaves with acidic fruits like rhubarb to sweeten the fruits.
Crystallizing: Add crystallized stems to desserts.

TIPS

Angelica dies after setting seeds; unless you're growing it for seeds, remove flowers early to prolong the life of the plant.

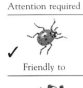
Attention required

Friendly to

Ornamental

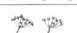
Container growing

Yield

Easy to grow

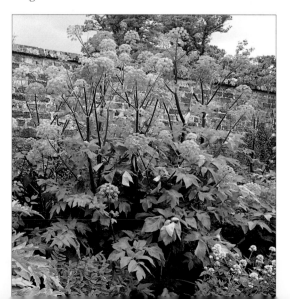

◀ **Angelica** *flowers give off a light, sweet fragrance, particularly in the early evening.*

Anise

Pimpinella anisum

Cakes, cookies, and breads made with licorice-flavored anise seeds are delicious! The sweetness of the seeds lets you cut down slightly on the sugar in your recipe, and you'll also appreciate the beneficial effect of anise on your digestive system.

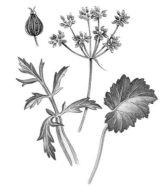

Attention required

 ✓
Friendly to

 ✓
Ornamental

✓
Container growing

Yield

Easy to grow

DESCRIPTION
Annual
2 feet tall; 1 to 2 feet wide
Flowers: Whitish yellow umbels, like those of Queen-Anne's-lace, bloom in summer.
Leaves: Anise's ferny leaves resemble those of Queen-Anne's-lace; plants have an airy habit.
Flavor and fragrance: Anise has a spicy sweet, licorice-like flavor and aroma.

▶ **Anise** *will self-seed in most gardens, giving you an almost perpetual patch.*

HOW TO GROW
When to plant: Sow seeds in spring where plants are to grow. Or start indoors in plantable peat or newspaper pots, eight weeks before your last spring frost date. Transplant to the garden after danger of frost is past.
Where to plant: Plant anise in full sun.
Soil and fertility: Anise grows best in light, lean, well-drained soil. Do not fertilize.

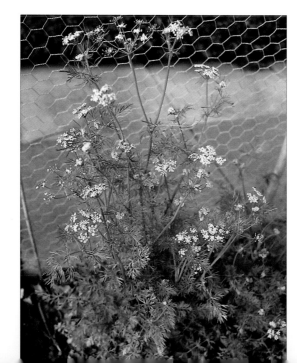

Plant spacing: Plant 1 foot apart in groups of five plants, or stake single plants to keep them upright.
Pests: Pest-free
Diseases: Disease-free

HARVESTING
When to harvest: Pick leaves in summer before plants bloom. Collect seeds when ripe at anytime when the dew is dry in early fall.
How to harvest: Snip leaves in the morning; for drying, strip leaves from cut stems. As seeds approach ripeness, enclose seed heads to prevent seeds from dropping. Cut whole seed heads when dew has dried.
Drying: Hang stems to air dry leaves. Let seeds dry fully, then store in tightly covered jars.
Freezing: Freeze chopped leaves.

USES
Cooking: Use fresh leaves and seeds in salads. Use dried, frozen, or fresh leaves with chicken, fish, and vegetables. Use seeds in baked goods and salads.
Medicinal: Anise aids digestion. Use a strong infusion of leaves or seeds to ease a cough.

TIPS
Anise is an excellent companion plant to cilantro.

Anise hyssop

Agastache foeniculum

Tasty as well as pretty, this ornamental herb is useful in teas, salads, and cooking. Enjoy anise hyssop's lovely purple blooms in the garden and in your flower arrangements.

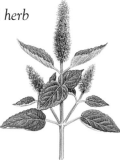

DESCRIPTION
Perennial
To 3 feet tall
Zones 5 to 9
Flowers: Spikes of lavender florets bloom from summer to fall.
Leaves: The mintlike leaves have toothed edges. Plants die back in winter.
Flavor and fragrance: Anise hyssop tastes and smells like "green" licorice.

HOW TO GROW
When to plant: Start indoors in plantable pots of peat or newspaper, eight weeks before your last spring frost date. Transplant to your garden after the last spring frost in your area. Or sow directly in the garden a week before your last spring frost date.
Where to plant: Prefers full sun but tolerates partial shade.
Soil and fertility: Plants grow best in moderately moist, well-drained soil that's high in fertility. Apply ½ inch of compost around base of plant each spring.

Plant spacing: Space plants 1 foot apart.
Pests: Usually pest-free
Diseases: Usually disease-free

HARVESTING
When to harvest: Harvest leaves for drying before the plant blooms; otherwise, harvest leaves anytime, gathering them in the morning. Cut flowers for drying when florets are three-quarters open.
How to harvest: Snip off leaves as needed, starting from the bottom of the plant. To dry for tea, cut whole stems about 4 to 5 inches from the base of the plant and strip the leaves off. Cut flowers with stems.
Drying: Hang upside down to air dry.

USES
Cooking: Fresh leaves are excellent in salads. Fresh and dried leaves make good teas, alone or in combination with other herbs. The licorice flavor of fresh minced leaves complements some fish and chicken dishes.

Medicinal: A strong tea aids digestion.
Arrangements: Use fresh or dried flowers in floral arrangements.

CULTIVARS AND RELATIVES
- Korean hyssop (*A. rugosa*) has a sharper flavor than anise hyssop.
- 'Snow Spike' (*A. foeniculum* 'Snow Spike'): white flowers.

TIPS
This plant is a favorite of bees and provides a good source of nectar in late summer and early fall. It repels cabbage moth.

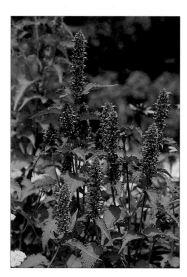

▲ **Anise hyssop**'s *lavender blooms are so lovely that you can always use extra plants in your flower gardens.*

Attention required

✓ Friendly to

✓ Ornamental

✓ Container growing

Yield

Easy to grow

Basil, sweet

Ocimum basilicum

Attention required

✓ Friendly to

✓ Ornamental

✓ Container growing

Yield

Easy to grow

No herb garden is complete without basil. With so many cultivars to choose from, it's fun to grow a sampler. This herb's rich history dates back to the civilizations of ancient Egypt, Greece, and Rome. Its Greek name, basilikon, means "royal."

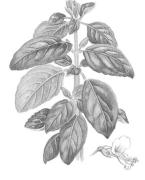

DESCRIPTION

Tender annual
Typically 1 to 2 feet tall; height varies according to cultivar
Flowers: Spikes of small white, pink, or purple florets bloom from midsummer to fall.
Leaves: Appearance depends on cultivar. Standard sweet basil has deep green, opposite, glossy leaves with smooth edges. The 'Ruffles' cultivars have frilled leaves with toothed edges. Anise basil (O. *basilicum* 'Anise') has green leaves with purple veins. Lemon basil (O. *basilicum* 'Americanum') has small, sharply pointed light green leaves with smooth edges. The leaves of East Indian basil (O. *gratissimum*) are covered with tiny gray hairs that make them look like soft felt.
Flavor and fragrance: Basil has a spicy-sweet flavor with undertones of pepper and, according to some palates, licorice. Its fragrance is strong, fresh, and pungent with hints of mint and pepper.

HOW TO GROW

When to plant: For earliest harvest, start basil seeds indoors, six weeks before your last spring frost date. Transplant to the garden after all danger of frost has passed. Make successive plantings, either directly in the garden or by transplanting seedlings, through July.
Where to plant: Basil prefers full sun.

Soil and fertility: Basil requires well-drained, moist, nutrient-rich soil. Till 1 inch of compost into the growing area before planting. Mulch with straw after the soil warms to retain high moisture levels.
Plant spacing: Space transplanted seedlings 12 to 18 inches apart. Thin direct-seeded crops as true leaves form.
Pests: Aphids, rose chafers, Japanese beetles, slugs
Diseases: In poorly drained soils and high humidity, fungal leaf spot diseases can occur. Fusarium wilt is increasingly common. Aphids can transmit cucumber mosaic virus.

▼ **'Purple Ruffles'** *basil not only tastes good, it's also an excellent ornamental.*

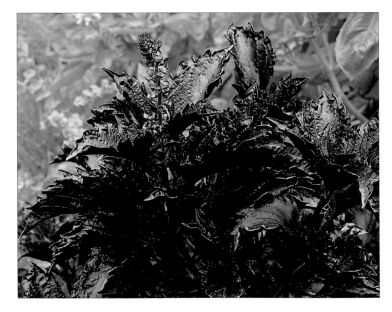

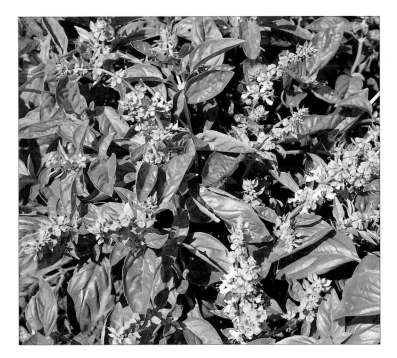

HARVESTING

When to harvest: Begin cutting leaves and stems when plants are 8 inches tall and before they bloom.

How to harvest: Harvest basil only when the leaves are dry. To promote bushiness, cut back the central stem, taking the top two or three sets of leaves. New branches will form in the axils where the leaves join the stem. Continue to pinch out branch tips, always leaving at least a pair of leaves below the cut so that new branches can form. Pinch or cut off flower spikes as soon as they form. For best quality, cut stems at internodes (between two leaves) and store harvested stems in a cool place, standing them in a jar of water.

Drying: Hang to air dry, but tastes better when frozen.

Freezing: Blanch leaves before freezing in ice cubes. Raw in butter or oil.

USES

Cooking: Use fresh, dried, or frozen with shellfish and in egg dishes, vegetable soups, pasta, salads, salad dressings, and entrees, particularly those containing tomatoes. Make into pesto.

Vinegars: Adds wonderful flavor to vinegars.

Oils: Combine with extra-virgin olive oil for flavored cooking oil.

Medicinal: Basil infusions promote digestion and may also reduce fevers. In the bath, basil acts as a stimulating herb.

Arrangements: Sprigs of basil add fragrance and beauty to fresh arrangements. Purple and ruffled-leaved cultivars are striking in arrangements.

———— ❧ ————

CULTIVARS AND RELATIVES

Many types of basil are available. These are some of the best:

- East Indian basil (*O. gratissimum*): Spicy, clovelike aroma and flavor; excellent with tomatoes and in curries.
- 'Genovese' (*O. basilicum* 'Genovese'): An excellent culinary basil, particularly good in pesto.
- 'Lemon' (*O. basilicum* 'Americanum'): Excellent for seasoning fish dishes and in salads.
- 'Lettuce-leaf' (*O. basilicum* 'Crispum'): Huge leaves, suitable for stuffing.
- 'Rubin' (*O. basilicum* 'Rubin'): Dark purple coloration with good flavor and fragrance.
- 'Spicy Globe' (*O. basilicum* 'Minimum'): Compact, rounded plant; tiny leaves have good flavor.
- West African basil (*O. viride*; *O. gratissimum*): Spicy flavor; used medicinally, as a gargle and dressing for wounds because of antiseptic qualities.

———— ❧ ————

TIPS

Basil repels many flying insects, so grace your picnic table with the potted herb or use freshly cut stems in a vase. Crush leaves to release their fragrance.

Bee balm

Monarda didyma

Bee balm, or Oswego tea, was the tea substitute of choice for American colonists who were boy-cotting black tea just before the Revolutionary War. Make some and you'll see how easy it was to hold the Boston Tea Party.

Attention required

Friendly to ✓

Ornamental ✓

Container growing ✗

Yield

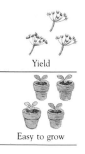

Easy to grow

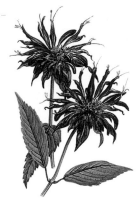

DESCRIPTION
Perennial
3 to 5 feet tall
Zones 3 to 9
Flowers: Tubular flowers bloom in showy tiered whorls at stem tips for several weeks in midsummer. Colors range from white to pink, purple, and red.
Leaves: Dark green, opposite leaves have toothed edges. Plants die back in winter.
Flavor and fragrance: Bee balm tastes and smells like mint with citrusy undertones.

HOW TO GROW
When to plant: Start seeds indoors eight weeks before the last spring frost date; transplant to the garden one week before the last spring frost. Divide plants or layer stems in early spring.
Where to plant: Bee balm prefers partial shade but tolerates full sun.
Soil and fertility: Plant in well-drained, moist, fertile soil. Apply ½ inch of compost each spring.
Plant spacing: Bee balm spreads rapidly. Give it at least 2 square feet of area initially. Mulch surrounding area heavily to help control its spreading, but be prepared to pull or dig out new sprouts.
Pests: Usually pest-free
Diseases: Rust; powdery mildew is common in late summer.

HARVESTING
When to harvest: Harvest small quantities of leaves anytime when the dew is dry. For drying in quantity, cut leaves before bloom in early summer and again in late August or early September. Cut flowers for drying when blooms are almost fully open.
How to harvest: Snip individual leaves or fresh flowers for salads. For drying in quantity, cut stems about 1 inch from the soil. For dried arrangements, cut stems at least 1 foot below the blossoms.
Drying: Strip leaves from stems

▶ **Bee balm** *always attracts hummingbirds.*

and dry them on screens or in a dehydrator. Hang flowers to dry.

USES
Cooking: Sprinkle fresh florets in salads. Fresh and dried leaves make good teas, alone or in combination with other herbs.
Arrangements and crafts: Use dried flowers to brighten potpourris. Add fresh or dried stems of flowers to arrangements.

CULTIVARS AND RELATIVES
- 'Cambridge Scarlet': Red blooms.
- 'Croftway Pink': Pink blooms.
- Lemon mint (*M. citriodora*): Pink-purple blooms.
- 'Marshall's Delight': Pink blooms; resistant to powdery mildew.
- Wild bergamot (*M. fistulosa*): Lavender flowers and a very strong fragrance.

TIPS
Bee balm is said to enhance the growth of tomatoes and peppers.

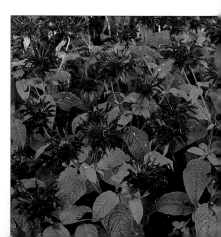

Betony

Stachys officinalis

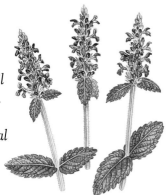

Betony had a powerful reputation during the Middle Ages and later: It was reputed to scare off any evil spirits that happened to be around. Today's herb gardeners appreciate betony as an interesting ornamental with a more practical medicinal history.

DESCRIPTION
Perennial
2 to 3 feet tall
Zones 4 to 8
Flowers: Tiered spikes of pinkish purple flowers bloom in midsummer.
Leaves: Bright green, opposite leaves have notched edges. Plants die back in winter.
Flavor and fragrance: Betony tastes and smells very similar to black tea.

HOW TO GROW
When to plant: Sow seeds indoors six to eight weeks before your last spring frost date; transplant to garden after your area's last spring frost. Or sow directly into the garden a week or two before the last spring frost. Divide plants every third year.
Where to plant: Betony prefers partial shade but will tolerate full sun.
Soil and fertility: Plant in well-drained, moderately moist soil of average fertility. Mulch with ½ inch of compost every other year.

Plant spacing: Space plants 12 to 18 inches apart; plants spread about 1 foot.
Pests: Largely pest-free
Diseases: Susceptible to root rot in soggy soils

HARVESTING
When to harvest: Harvest leaves before plant blooms in early July. For best quality, gather in the morning when the dew is dry.
How to harvest: Cut stems several inches above soil line and strip the leaves off.
Drying: Hang upside down to air dry.

USES
Cooking: Betony tastes like black tea but contains no caffeine.
Medicinal: Betony is said to relieve headaches brought on by tension and also contains tannins that can ease throat irritations and diarrhea. Excessive internal use irritates the stomach.

CULTIVARS AND RELATIVES
- Lamb's-ears (*S. byzantina*): A popular ornamental ground-cover with gray woolly leaves and soft lavender flowers.
- 'Primrose Heron' (*S. byzantina* 'Primrose Heron'): Pale yellow flowers.
- 'Silver Carpet' (*S. byzantina* 'Silver Carpet'): Rarely blooms and is grown for its fuzzy soft silver foliage.

TIPS
Betony makes an attractive addition to the perennial border.

▼ **Betony** *flowers bring a touch of color – and visiting bees – to the herb garden.*

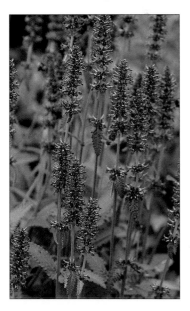

Attention required

✓ Friendly to

✓ Ornamental

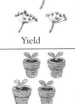
✓ Container growing

Yield

Easy to grow

Borage

Borago officinalis

Grow borage for its clear blue flowers and its cool, cucumbery flavor. Borage is said to strengthen the pest and disease resistance of plants growing around it, particularly strawberries. Bees love borage and are attracted to gardens where it blooms.

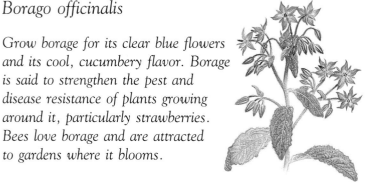

Attention required

 ✓
Friendly to

 ✓
Ornamental

 ✓
Container growing

Yield

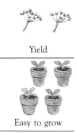
Easy to grow

DESCRIPTION

Annual

3 feet tall

Flowers: Clear blue, star-shaped flowers about ¾ inch in diameter bloom in drooping clusters from midsummer to frost. Each flower has interesting black anthers at its cone-shaped center.

Leaves: Broad, hairy leaves have prominent veins. The plant forms a rosette when young. Leaves on the upper portion of plant are alternate and up to 6 inches long.

Flavor and fragrance: Borage leaves and flowers have a salty, close-to-cucumber taste.

HOW TO GROW

When to plant: Sow in peat or newspaper pots six to eight weeks before your last spring frost date. Transplant seedlings to the garden or direct-sow seeds after the danger of frost has passed.

Where to plant: Borage prefers full sun but tolerates partial shade, particularly in southern areas. Plants generally do best in cool temperatures.

Soil and fertility: Plant in moist, fertile, well-drained soil.

Plant spacing: Allow 2 square feet per plant.

Pests: Usually pest-free

Diseases: Susceptible to root rot in soggy soils

HARVESTING

When to harvest: Harvest leaves at anytime in the growing season, gathering them in the morning when the dew has dried. Pick flowers when they're fully open in the morning when quite dry.

How to harvest: Snip individual leaves or strip off cut stems. Snip individual flowers or pinch off entire clusters.

Freezing: Freeze borage flowers in ice cubes for a decorative touch in iced drinks.

▶ **Borage** *fairly drips with starry blue flowers from summer to fall. The tall plants add a majestic touch to any garden.*

USES

Cooking: Borage has a flavor similar to cucumber. Mince leaves in yogurt or snip them over soups, salads, curries, fish, and chicken dishes. Steam leaves to eat as a vegetable. Add fresh flowers to salads.

Vinegars: Use leaves to make a lightly flavored vinegar.

Crystallizing: Crystallize flowers for decorations on pastries.

Medicinal: Borage leaf tea is said to be slightly laxative in action.

TIPS

Borage is a favorite bee food and provides nectar from mid-season to fall. This plant self-seeds easily, so be prepared to transplant and give away volunteers.

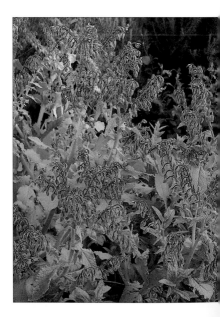

Calendula

Calendula officinalis

Romans named calendula in honor of the plant's ability to bloom on the first day of every month – in the right climate, that is. In northern areas, you'll have to wait until midsummer for its vividly colored flowers.

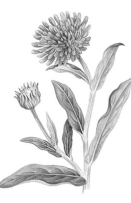

DESCRIPTION

Annual

18 inches tall

Flowers: Bright yellow or orange daisylike flowers bloom from midsummer to after frost. Flowers close at dusk.

Leaves: Oblong or oval leaves have smooth edges and a prominent middle vein. The upper leaves clasp the stalk.

Flavor and fragrance: Calendula petals do not have a particularly strong flavor or fragrance. They are typically used in salad mixes to add color rather than flavor.

HOW TO GROW

When to plant: In Zone 5 or colder, start seeds indoors about eight weeks before your last spring frost date; transplant seedlings to the garden a week or two before that date. Or, in Zones 5 to 6, plant seeds outside after the soil has warmed to 60°F. In Zones 7 to 9, sow seeds in fall, where they are to grow.

Where to plant: Calendula prefers full sun in the North and partial shade in the South. Intolerant of intense heat.

Soil and fertility: Plant in fertile, moist, well-drained soil.

Plant spacing: Space plants 8 to 10 inches apart.

Pests: Slugs, snails, aphids, thrips

Diseases: Susceptible to many, including leaf spot, stem rot, downy mildew, powdery mildew

HARVESTING

When to harvest: Harvest flowers just after they open fully throughout spring and summer, gathering them in the morning when the dew is dry.

How to harvest: Cut stem at the joint nearest to the flower.

Drying: Separate petals and lay on parchment paper in a dehydrator or between sheets of brown paper in the shade. Keep petals from touching each other or they may discolor. Store in an airtight container in a dark, dry location.

USES

Cooking: Add fresh petals to salads and sprinkle over green vegetables. Use dried petals for coloring cooked rice.

Cosmetic: Use calendula flowers in massage oils and salves to soften skin. Makes a conditioner for oily hair and gives hair body.

Crafts: Add dried petals to potpourris for visual appeal.

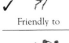

Attention required

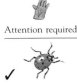
✓

Friendly to

✓

Ornamental

✓

Container growing

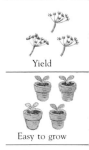

Yield

Easy to grow

◀ **Calendula** *will flower with the last mums if you make a second planting in mid-July.*

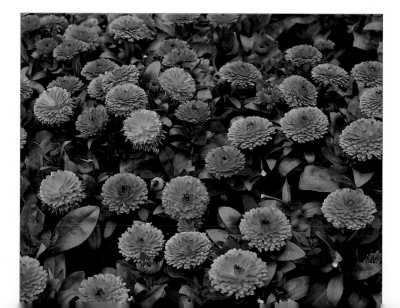

Caraway

Carum carvi

Caraway has one of the oldest histories of all the herbs. It's been found in meals left behind in dwellings from the Stone Age, and Egyptians included it in the supplies packed in the tombs of their pharaohs.

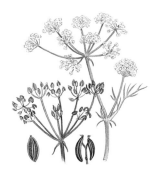

DESCRIPTION

Annual or biennial
Annuals to 2 feet; biennials to 8 inches in first year, to 2 feet in second year
Zones 3 to 9
Flowers: Flat, Queen-Anne's-lace-like umbels of tiny white flowers bloom in late summer. Biennial cultivars bloom in their second year.
Leaves: The ferny green leaves resemble those of carrots. Biennials die back under severe cold during the winter but sprout again the second spring.
Flavor and fragrance: Caraway seeds and roots have a sharp, spicy taste and fragrance, while the leaves taste like those of dill.

HOW TO GROW

When to plant: Sow in the garden as soon as the soil can be worked in spring.
Where to plant: Prefers full sun but will tolerate partial shade in southern regions.
Soil and fertility: Caraway prefers sandy, well-drained, slightly dry soils; however, the

plant will suffer if the surface of the soil dries out below the first inch or so. Scratch ½ inch of compost into the first couple of inches of soil before planting.
Plant spacing: Space plants 6 to 8 inches apart.
Pests: Aphids, carrot weevils
Diseases: Crown rot

HARVESTING

When to harvest: Harvest leaves anytime after the plant is 5 to 6 inches tall. Harvest seeds when they are ripe. Gather both leaves and seeds only when completely dry. Harvest roots in the fall.
How to harvest: Cut leaf stems at their base or strip off cut stems. When seed heads begin ripening, enclose them in a paper sack or in a swatch of floating row cover material to catch seeds that might fall, and cut off entire seed head.

▶ **Caraway** *reseeds so easily that you may get a "permanent" patch that you have to thin or transplant from every year.*

USES

Cooking: Use fresh leaves in soups, stews, and salads and as a garnish. Add seeds to breads, salad dressings, and German and Scandinavian dishes. The flavor complements cabbage, beets, potatoes, beans, cheeses, eggs, and meats. Steam roots and eat them like parsnips.
Medicinal: A mild infusion made by steeping crushed caraway seeds in water or milk may be used as a tonic for digestive upset.

TIPS

In cold climates, mulch plants well for the winter if they have not flowered the first season.

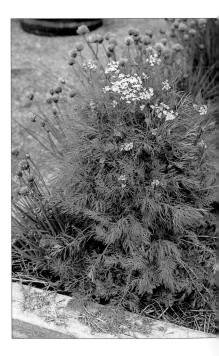

Catnip

Nepeta cataria

Imagine your cat's pleasure when you plant this herb. If you dry a good supply, you'll have enough to make catnip toys for all the cats you know and catnip tea for their grateful owners.

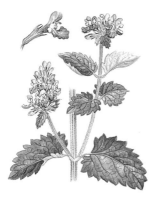

DESCRIPTION
Perennial
2 to 3 feet tall
Zones 3 to 9
Flowers: Spikes of pinkish purple or white flowers bloom in midsummer.
Leaves: Leaves are opposite with toothed margins and heart-shaped bases, about 2 to 3 inches long. Both stems and leaves are covered with downy soft hairs. Plants die back over the winter months.
Flavor and fragrance: In teas, catnip has a flavor that is more mellow than peppermint and less sweet than spearmint. Its fragrance is spicy-minty.

HOW TO GROW
When to plant: Sow seeds in the garden about two weeks before your last spring frost date.
Where to plant: In northern areas, plant in full sun. In the South, plant in partial shade or in moist soil in full sun.
Soil and fertility: Catnip prefers moist, well-drained soils of average fertility. Scratch ½ inch of compost into the top few inches of soil before planting, and side-dress with compost every spring.
Plant spacing: Space plants 8 to 10 inches apart.
Pests: Catnip rarely suffers from insect pests, but cats may nibble its leaves and can crush young plants.
Diseases: Anthracnose, rust, root rot

HARVESTING
When to harvest: Snip leaves anytime, gathering them in the morning when the dew is dry; the flavor is milder before the plant blooms. If harvesting for medicinal uses or for your cats, wait until the plant blooms.
How to harvest: Snip off individual leaves. When harvesting to dry, cut whole stems, complete with flowerstalks, about 2 inches from the soil surface.
Drying: Hang upside down to air dry, or strip leaves and flowers from stems and dry in a dehydrator.

USES
Cooking: Catnip was once a common ingredient in salads. Snip in a few leaves to see if the taste appeals to you. Otherwise, make teas from fresh or dried leaves.
Medicinal: Try tea made from the dried leaves and flowers of catnip as an after-dinner aid to digestion or a before-bedtime sleep inducer.
Crafts: Catnip toys are a favorite with cats.

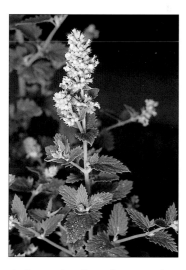

▲ **Catnip**'s *velvety leaves and mounded growth habit make it a good plant to use as a background for smaller herbs.*

TIPS
Keep your catnip safe from cats by enclosing it in a sturdy chicken-wire cage until it's well established.

Attention required

✓ Friendly to

✓ Ornamental

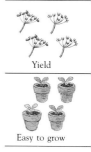
✓ Container growing

Yield

Easy to grow

Chamomile

Matricaria recutita, German chamomile
Chamaemelum nobile, Roman chamomile

Attention required

 ✓
Friendly to

✓
Ornamental

✓
Container growing

Yield

Easy to grow

Teas made from homegrown, freshly picked and dried chamomile flowers taste so much better than store-bought that you're likely to make this plant a permanent feature of your herb garden.

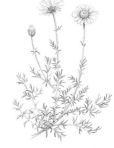

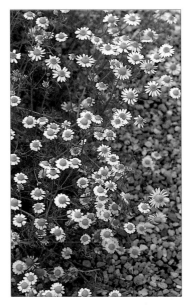

▲ **Chamomile**'s *bountiful flowers are soothing when dried and used to make tea.*

DESCRIPTION

German chamomile
Annual
2 to 3 feet tall

Roman chamomile
Perennial
8 to 10 inches tall
Zones 5 to 9

Flowers: Both chamomiles have daisylike flowers with yellow centers surrounded by whitish petals.

Leaves: German chamomile is an erect plant with feathery-looking leaves covered with soft hairs. Roman chamomile has creeping stems and somewhat coarser leaves.

Flavor and fragrance: In teas, the fresh, clean flavor of chamomile is immediately soothing. Its fragrance is similar to that of freshly cut hay.

HOW TO GROW

When to plant: Sow both types of chamomile in the garden when soil temperatures have reached 55° to 60°F.

Where to plant: Both chamomiles prefer full sun but will tolerate partial shade.

Soil and fertility: Well-drained sandy soils with moderate fertility levels are ideal for German chamomile; if your soil is moist, plant in a raised bed. Roman chamomile prefers a rich, moist soil. Scratch in ½ inch of compost to the top few

inches of soil before planting Roman chamomile, and apply the same amount as a topdressing every spring.

Plant spacing: Allow 6 to 8 inches between German chamomile plants and 18 inches between Roman chamomile plants.

Pests: Both are pest-free.

Diseases: Both are disease-free.

HARVESTING

When to harvest: When flowers are fully open which will be late spring and summer for German chamomile and slightly earlier for Roman chamomile.

How to harvest: Cut whole stems of German chamomile. Pinch off the flowers of Roman chamomile.

Drying: Dry on screens.

USES

Teas: Both chamomiles make excellent teas.

Medicinal: Teas are said to be sleep inducing. People who have known sensitivities to ragweed may also suffer allergic reactions to chamomile.

Cosmetic: Make rinses and conditioners to heighten blonde highlights, help prevent dandruff, and condition dry hair. Cosmetic preparations containing chamomile are also used to soften the skin and refresh the eyes.

Crafts: Add chamomile flowers to potpourris.

Chervil

Anthriscus cerefolium

Chervil's subtle, warming flavor is so good that the more you use it, the more uses you'll find for it. If this herb is new to you, plant a small patch and give it a try.

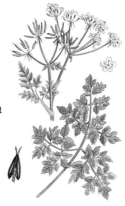

DESCRIPTION
Annual
12 to 18 inches tall
Flowers: Tiny white flowers bloom in Queen-Anne's-lace-like umbels in early summer.
Leaves: The green ferny leaves resemble those of carrots.
Flavor and fragrance: Chervil's flavor is like a mixture of mild licorice and young parsley leaves; it has a delicate fragrance.

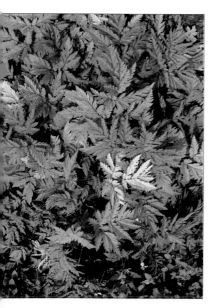

HOW TO GROW
When to plant: Sow in a bed of very fine soil or sprinkle seeds over a layer of fine vermiculite about a week or two before your last spring frost date. Make a second planting in mid- to late summer.
Where to plant: In the North, plant spring crops in full sun. In southern areas and for second plantings in the North, choose a location with filtered shade. Chervil is intolerant of heat and will bolt (flower and set seed) prematurely if exposed to high temperatures.
Soil and fertility: Plants require rich, moist soil. Apply ½ inch of compost to planting area before seeding.
Plant spacing: Space plants 6 to 8 inches apart.
Pests: Aphids, carrot weevils
Diseases: Occasionally develops leaf spot when temperatures

◀ **Chervil**'s *delicate flavor is a popular feature of French cuisine.*

and humidity are high. Plant in raised beds to improve drainage and air circulation.

HARVESTING
When to harvest: Begin harvesting leaves when plants are 6 inches tall. Gather the leaves in the morning throughout the summer before the plant blooms.
How to harvest: Cut outside stems at a node (where leaf or branch attaches to stem). Pinch out flowerstalks to prolong harvest period.
Freezing: Freeze in butter or ice cubes.

USES
Cooking: Use chervil in soups, stews, salads, potato dishes, sprinkled over pork, fish and egg dishes, and cooked beans and peas, and any other foods in which you would use parsley. Mince fresh leaves for salads. Add leaves to cooked dishes just before serving so that they don't lose their flavor.
Oils: Combine with extra-virgin olive oil or saffron or canola oil for flavored cooking oil.

TIPS
Plant chervil every two weeks through the growing season in a location with partial shade to have a continuous supply of leaves. Chervil self-sows, providing you with a bonus crop.

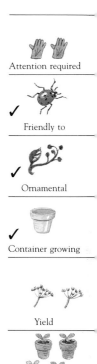

Attention required

✓ Friendly to

✓ Ornamental

✓ Container growing

Yield

Easy to grow

Chives

Allium schoenoprasum, chives
A. tuberosum, garlic chives

Chives at your own back door offer fresh oniony greens from early spring through the fall. Sprinkle snipped leaves over everything from stir-fry to scrambled eggs. Add the pretty purple flowers to vinegars and salads.

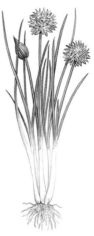

Attention required

✓
Friendly to

✓
Ornamental

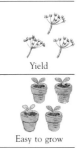
✓
Container growing

Yield

Easy to grow

DESCRIPTION

Perennials
12 to 18 inches tall
Zones 3 to 10

Flowers: Chives has globe-shaped clusters of pink to purple florets in mid-spring. Garlic chives bears loose clusters of star-shaped white or mauve florets in late summer.

Leaves: Chives has hollow, cylindrical leaves; garlic chives has flat leaves. Both die back in the fall.

Flavor and fragrance: Chives has an oniony flavor and fragrance; garlic chives tastes and smells like mild garlic.

HOW TO GROW

When to plant: Sow directly in the garden in early spring, or start seeds indoors at least eight weeks before your last spring frost date. Seeds require darkness to germinate. Transplant seedlings anytime from early spring to late summer. Protect new transplants from late spring frosts. Divide chives every three years to prevent overcrowding. In early spring or early fall, dig the clump with a spade. Trim the roots to about 3 inches long and the tops to about 2 inches long. Gently pull the clump into sections of four to six bulbs each. Replant these sections 8 to 12 inches apart in a row.

Where to plant: Plant chives in full sun to partial shade.

Soil and fertility: Both types require well-drained, humus-rich soils. Before planting, till 1 inch of compost into the growing area. Apply ½ inch of compost to the soil surface around the plants during mid-summer. After the leaves die back in the fall, apply ½ inch of compost to the entire growing bed.

Plant spacing: Space groups of four to six seedlings 8 to 12 inches apart. Direct-sow seeds in groups at the same spacing to make early weeding easy.

Pests: Few problems

Diseases: In soggy soils and high humidity, crowded plants can develop fungal diseases.

HARVESTING

When to harvest: Harvest after leaves are at least 6 inches tall.

How to harvest: Cut leaves with a sharp knife or shears at least 2 inches above the soil. Snip off flowers just after they open fully, removing all flowerstalks. Cut back chives after flowering.

Drying: Home-dried chives usually lack color and flavor.

Freezing: Freeze in ice cubes.

USES

Cooking: Snip leaves into salads, soups, and egg dishes. Sprinkle over cooked fish and other entrees to add flavor and a fresh appearance. Toss whole flower clusters or florets into salads.

Vinegars: Use in vinegars for a light, oniony flavor.

Oils: Combine with extra-virgin olive oil.

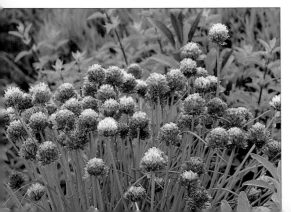

◄ **Chives** *are so tasty and so easy to grow that you'll soon find yourself snipping a few leaves to add to almost every meal.*

Cilantro/Coriander

Coriandrum sativum

Don't stop at salsa when you sample your cilantro! Snip fresh leaves into soups, salads, East Indian curries and dahls, and South and Central American dishes. It complements all these flavors and more.

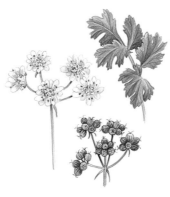

DESCRIPTION
Annual
2 to 3 feet tall
Flowers: Flat white to pinkish umbels that resemble parsley flowers bloom about three to four months after sowing.
Leaves: The ferny leaves resemble those of flat-leaved parsley or Queen-Anne's-lace.
Flavor and fragrance: Cilantro leaves have a sharp "green" flavor and aroma. The seeds are sweet and spicy in both flavor and fragrance.

HOW TO GROW
When to plant: Cilantro does not transplant well. Start in plantable peat or newspaper pots about six weeks before your last spring frost date, or sow directly in the garden after that date. Make successive plantings every month thereafter until early August.
Where to plant: Plant in full sun in northern areas and for spring plantings; partial or filtered shade in the South and for summer plantings.
Soil and fertility: Cilantro prefers well-drained moist soil of moderate fertility. Too much nitrogen diminishes flavor.
Plant spacing: Space plants 8 to 10 inches apart.
Pests: Usually pest-free
Diseases: Susceptible to root rot and leaf spot in poorly drained soils

HARVESTING
When to harvest: Harvest leaves when plants are 5 to 6 inches tall. Gather leaves in the morning in spring and summer before the plant blooms. Harvest seeds (called coriander) when dry and fully ripe, summer through fall.
How to harvest: Cut off leaf stems at a node (where leaf attaches to stem), taking outside leaves first. Enclose ripening seed heads to prevent them from dropping seeds onto the ground, and remove entire seed head.

▶ **Cilantro** *was almost unknown in the U.S. until salsa became popular.*

Freezing: Freeze leaves in ice cubes or butter.

USES
Cooking: Cilantro leaves (fresh, dried, or frozen) are vital in salsa and many other tomato sauces, particularly those made for Mexican, Asian, or East Indian dishes, and with cooked beans, rice, fish, and poultry. Use fresh leaves in salads. Use seeds in curries and with fish, poultry, and legumes.
Oils: Combine with extra-virgin olive oil or saffron or canola oil for flavored cooking oil.
Crafts: Add coriander seeds to potpourris for fragrance.

TIPS
Cilantro self-sows easily, giving you a second crop during most seasons and a repeat crop in the following year. Pinch off stems with buds for bushy growth and to limit self-sowing.

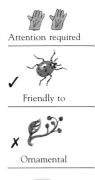
Attention required

✓ Friendly to

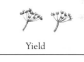
✗ Ornamental

✓ Container growing

Yield

Easy to grow

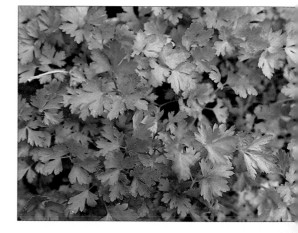

Clary

Salvia sclarea

Clary is lovely enough to grow for its looks alone. But it's useful, too, in everything from infusions for skin care to potpourris and poultry seasoning.

Attention required

Friendly to ✓

Ornamental ✓

Container growing ✓

Yield

Easy to grow

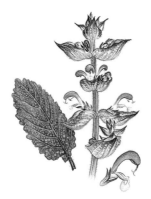

DESCRIPTION
Biennial
2½ to 3 feet tall
Zones 4 to 7
Flowers: Pink to purple-blue or white bracts surround the small flowers, which grow in spikes, blooming in mid- to late summer.
Leaves: The gray-green opposite leaves are wrinkled and downy with slightly toothed edges.
Flavor and fragrance: Clary, also called clary sage, tastes much like culinary sage and has a warm, pungent fragrance with a hint of camphor. The leaves can be bitter if used in too great a quantity.

HOW TO GROW
When to plant: Freeze seeds for three to five days before planting. Seeds require darkness for germination. Start seeds indoors about eight weeks before your last spring frost date. Transplant seedlings to the garden about one week before that date. Direct-sow in the garden once the soil has warmed to 55° to 60°F.

Where to plant: Plant clary in full sun.
Soil and fertility: Clary grows best in well-drained, somewhat sandy soil, of average fertility. Do not fertilize with high nitrogen materials. Allow the top inch or two of soil to dry between waterings.
Plant spacing: Space plants 9 to 12 inches apart.
Pests: Two-spotted spider mites
Diseases: Susceptible to root rot in poorly drained soil

HARVESTING
When to harvest: Pick leaves in the morning when the dew is dry at anytime in the growing season. Cut flowering stems once the flowers are three-quarters open.
How to harvest: Snip leaves when needed, or strip off cut stems. Cut whole stems of flowers near the base of the plant.
Drying: Hang upside down to air dry.

USES
Cooking: Clary sage tastes just like culinary sage. Use it fresh

or dried interchangeably to season breads, stuffings, cheese dishes, and vegetables.
Medicinal: A strong infusion of the crushed seeds is sometimes used as an eyewash. You can also add an infusion of the leaves to bathwater for a stimulating soak.
Arrangements and crafts: Wonderful in fresh or dried floral arrangements. Use the flowers in potpourri, particularly in combination with lavender and bee balm.

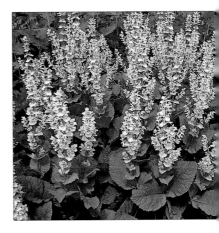

▲ **Clary** *in bloom makes such a good show that it rivals all the other ornamental salvias.*

TIPS
After the first frost, cut the stems of first-year plants to 1 inch above the soil. Mulch heavily to protect the roots over the winter. Clary self-seeds quite easily. Transplant or pull out unwanted volunteers.

Comfrey

Symphytum officinale

Comfrey leaves are good medicine for the potato crop: Use the leaves as a mulch over your potato hills, and potassium and other minerals will leach out to feed the spuds.

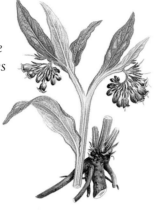

DESCRIPTION
Perennial
3 to 5 feet tall; 3 to 4 feet wide
Zones 3 to 9
Flowers: Drooping racemes of ½-inch-long tubular flowers in colors ranging from blue to yellow and cream bloom in late spring through summer.
Leaves: Comfrey's large, hairy, oval leaves have prominent veins and smooth edges.
Flavor and fragrance: Not applicable – do not eat.

HOW TO GROW
When to plant: Plant root divisions in early spring in the North and early fall in the South.
Where to plant: Comfrey prefers full sun but will tolerate partial shade.
Soil and fertility: Plant in moist fertile soil. Comfrey is tough enough to take less than ideal soil drainage but prefers well-drained areas.
Plant spacing: Allow 3 square feet per plant.
Pests: Pest-free
Diseases: Largely disease-free

HARVESTING
When to harvest: Pick young leaves during the spring and early summer, gathering them in the morning when the dew is dry. Harvest comfrey roots in the fall after the plant begins to die back, choosing a dry day and leaving some rootstock remaining.
How to harvest: Snip off leaves as needed or strip from cut stems. Dig roots and cut off only the smaller rhizomes that grow from the sides of the central root. Replant the central root.
Drying: Dry leaves flat on screens. Cut rhizomes into 1- to 2-inch pieces and dry in a dehydrator.

USES
Medicinal: Comfrey is a suspected carcinogen and should never be taken internally. However, a tincture or infusion of comfrey leaves or roots promotes healing of surface wounds, burns, and bruises. The active ingredient, allantoin, is added to many skin care medications. A decoction of comfrey root is useful for stopping the bleeding from a minor cut.
Cosmetic: Makes a conditioner for dry hair.

CULTIVARS AND RELATIVES
● Russian comfrey (*S. × uplandicum*): Similar to *S. officinale* but without the medicinal qualities of true comfrey.

TIPS
Comfrey is almost impossible to eliminate once it is established. Plant it only where it can live for many years. To eradicate it, be persistent about digging sprouts and all the roots you can find through the spring and early summer. Then mulch with a foot of organic material covered with layers of black plastic until fall.

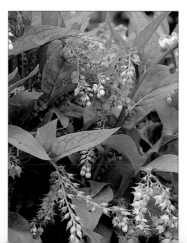

◄ **Comfrey** *needs a permanent site where its invasive nature won't disturb other plants.*

Attention required

✓ Friendly to

✓ Ornamental

✓ Container growing

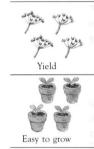
Yield

Easy to grow

Dill

Anethum graveolens

Dilly beans, dilled yogurt, dilled cheese sauces – the ferny leaves of this herb add a tang of flavor to all kinds of dishes. Plant small patches all through the summer for a steady supply.

Attention required

  ✓
Friendly to

✓
Ornamental

  ✓
Container growing

Yield

Easy to grow

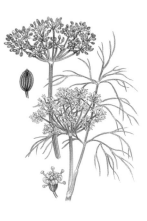

DESCRIPTION
Annual
1½ to 5 feet tall, depending on cultivar
Flowers: Flat umbels about 6 inches across with many tiny yellowish flowers bloom three to four months after sowing.
Leaves: Dill has ferny, threadlike blue-green foliage.
Flavor and fragrance: Dill leaves have a spicy, slightly sharp flavor and fragrance. The seeds have a sharper flavor that is almost bitter.

HOW TO GROW
When to plant: Sow directly in the garden after your last spring

frost date. To get an early start, sow four or five seeds per peat pot five weeks before your last spring frost date and transplant the pots at a 12-inch spacing in the row. Make a second planting of dill in early July for a continuous supply.
Where to plant: Plant dill in full sun.
Soil and fertility: Plants grow best in moist, well-drained fertile soil.
Plant spacing: Allow 6 to 8 inches between plants.
Pests: Largely pest-free
Diseases: Generally disease-free

HARVESTING
When to harvest: Cut leaves after plants are about 6 inches tall, gathering them in the morning when the dew is dry, summer to early fall. Cut leaves for drying just before the plant

blooms. Collect seed heads for pickles from the time the flowers are fully open to just before the seeds ripen. Harvest ripe seeds for drying.
How to harvest: Snip off individual leaves when plants are young. Cut whole stems of foliage for drying, and strip the leaves off. For use in pickles, cut off seed heads with an inch or so of stem attached. Enclose seed head before it turns brown, and remove whole head.
Drying: Hang stems upside down to dry foliage, or cut into small pieces and dry on the fruit leather insert of a dehydrator. Strip dried leaves from the stems. To dry seeds, enclose seed heads in a paper bag or cheesecloth and hang the stems upside down.
Freezing: Freeze leaves in ice cubes.

USES
Cooking: Use leaves or seeds to flavor soups, cheeses, fish, beef, poultry, and egg, bean, pea, and vegetable dishes. Dill complements almost all cabbage-family vegetables. It is also tasty used fresh in green salads, with sliced tomatoes and cucumbers, and in potato salad.
Vinegars: Use in vinegars for tangy flavor.
Oils: Combine with extra-virgin olive oil or saffron or canola oil.
Arrangements: Use the flower umbels in fresh bouquets.

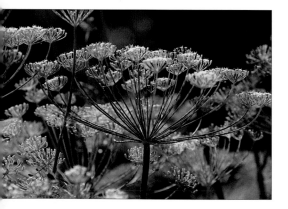

◄ **Dill**'s *clusters of tiny flowers attract bees and other beneficials to the garden. Cut or enclose seed heads before they ripen to limit self-sowing.*

Fennel

Foeniculum vulgare

The lacy leaves of fennel are a beautiful addition to the perennial border. Clip a few stems and mix them with nasturtiums and calendula to create an attractive and edible centerpiece for the table.

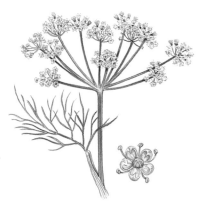

DESCRIPTION

Perennial grown as annual, except in southernmost areas
2 to 5 feet tall
Zones 6 to 9
Flowers: The 6-inch-wide umbels of tiny yellow flowers appear in midsummer.
Leaves: Fennel's feathery, blue-green leaves look remarkably like those of dill.
Flavor and fragrance: Fennel leaves and seeds have a mild licorice or anise flavor and fragrance.

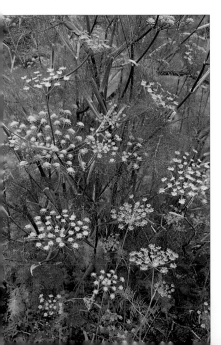

HOW TO GROW

When to plant: Sow directly in the garden a week or two before your last spring frost date. South of Zone 5, you can also plant fennel seeds in fall.
Where to plant: Prefers full sun but tolerates partial shade, particularly in southern areas.
Soil and fertility: Fennel requires moderately fertile, well-drained, moist soil, but will not tolerate overwatering.
Plant spacing: Space plants 6 inches apart.
Pests: Largely pest-free
Diseases: Prone to root rot in soggy soils

HARVESTING

When to harvest: Harvest leaves before the plant blooms, gathering them in the morning when the dew is dry. Collect ripe seeds on a dry day.
How to harvest: Snip individual leaves as needed. To

◄ **Fennel** *in your garden helps to repel pesky slugs and snails.*

harvest leaves for drying, cut whole stems. Enclose ripening seed heads in paper bags to prevent seeds from shattering onto the ground, and remove whole seed head.
Drying: Hang stems of leaves upside down to air dry. Hang flower stems upside down with the seed head enclosed.
Freezing: Freeze leaves in ice cubes.

USES

Cooking: Snip fresh leaves or mince stems into salads or over fish, pork, eggs, cheese, beans, rice, and cabbage-family vegetables. Add seeds to Asian dishes, sauerkraut, fish, lentils, breads, butter, and cheese spreads. Fennel's flavor fades quickly when heated; add it to recipes just before serving.
Oils: Combine with extra-virgin olive oil or saffron or canola oil for flavored cooking oil.
Medicinal: A fennel infusion aids digestion and reduces colic in infants and flatulence in children and adults.
Cosmetic: You can use fennel seeds to exfoliate dead skin and refine pores.
Arrangements: Use fresh fennel flowers in floral arrangements.

TIPS

Fennel seeds contain a volatile oil that produces an allergic reaction in some people who touch them.

Attention required

✓

Friendly to

✓

Ornamental

✓

Container growing

Yield

Easy to grow

Feverfew

Chrysanthemum parthenium

Feverfew masquerades as a fresh white daisy in the perennial border. But once you begin nibbling on it, you'll find that it really is a useful medicinal herb.

Attention required

　✗
Friendly to

　✓
Ornamental

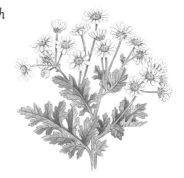

DESCRIPTION

Perennial
2 feet tall
Zones 5 to 7
Flowers: Numerous small white daisylike flowers with golden centers bloom from midsummer to early fall.
Leaves: The light green to golden green leaves are deeply lobed and divided into three segments; they generally grow up to 3 inches long. Plants die back during the winter months.
Flavor and fragrance: Feverfew has a bitter flavor and aroma.

HOW TO GROW

When to plant: Sow indoors about eight weeks before your last spring frost date and transplant to the garden a week or two after that date. South of Zone 5, plant directly in the garden once soil temperatures have reached 60°F. Divide in spring; take root divisions with some stem in early fall.
Where to plant: Feverfew prefers full sun but tolerates partial or filtered shade.
Soil and fertility: Plant in well-drained soils with average fertility. Excess nitrogen reduces flower production.
Plant spacing: Space plants 12 inches apart.
Pests: Aphids
Diseases: Susceptible to root rot in soggy soils

◀ **Feverfew** *self-sows readily enough to become a weed in the garden. Let it spread if you want more, or remove spent flowers to keep it in bounds.*

HARVESTING

When to harvest: Harvest leaves in the morning when the dew has dried. Pick leaves to dry for medicinal use before plant blooms. Cut flowers for fresh or dried arrangements in dry weather, when the blooms are three-quarters open.
How to harvest: Snip off individual leaves. Cut whole stems, an inch or so above the soil surface, for drying.
Drying: Hang stems upside down to air dry.
Freezing: Freeze leaves in ice cubes.

USES

Medicinal: Infusions of feverfew have been shown to reduce the frequency and severity of migraine headaches. Simply eating no more than three or four fresh leaves a day also has this effect. Because they taste bitter, you may want to drizzle honey on them to mask the flavor. Feverfew leaves also give relief from arthritis pain and impart calm and well-being.
Arrangements: Use feverfew flowers in fresh arrangements or dry them for winter bouquets.

TIPS

Bees dislike the odor of feverfew pollen and will steer clear of it; leave at least 20 feet between feverfew and any flowers, such as raspberries, that bloom at the same time and require pollination.

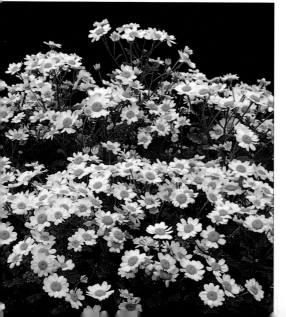

Geraniums, scented

Pelargonium spp.

A group of scented geraniums is irresistible on the patio table, in the garden, by the doorstep – everywhere. Collecting these wonderfully fragrant plants is one of the true joys of herb gardening.

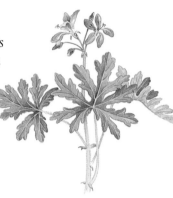

DESCRIPTION

Perennials, grown as annuals in cooler zones
1 to 3 feet tall, depending on species
Zone 10
Flowers: Not nearly as flashy as common bedding geraniums, these plants have open clusters of usually pale pink or white flowers. The upper two petals are usually larger than the lower three and are often a different color. Most species that are kept indoors all winter will bloom in late winter. Plants kept outdoors bloom in summer.
Leaves: Scented geraniums offer a wonderful variety of leaf shapes and textures. Some are dainty and scalloped, others broad and lobed, or lacy, crinkled, or curled, in all shades of green and gray-green.
Flavor and fragrance: The flavor of scented geraniums is somewhat sweet and refreshing at the same time. Fragrance varies remarkably with different species and cultivars – scented geraniums can smell like spicy roses, lemons, apples, or even pineapples.

HOW TO GROW

When to plant: Plant in your garden or move containers outdoors after all danger of frost is past and night temperatures are 50°F or higher. Scented geraniums are best started from cuttings or young plants, but seeds are available for apple, coconut, and peppermint geraniums. Seeds are slow to germinate. Sow seeds in a flat and keep on a heated mat at 80°F; prick out individual seedlings as they sprout and transplant them into small individual pots. Allow at least three months for seeds to germinate.
Where to plant: Plants prefer full sun but tolerate the filtered

▶ **Scented geraniums** *that are overwintered indoors often bloom as early as February.*

light of a south windowsill.
Soil and fertility: Pot in a humus-rich medium and keep moist.
Plant spacing: Space plants 12 inches apart. Pot cuttings in 4-inch containers and move up as the plants grow. A fully mature scented geranium will fill a 12-inch pot.
Pests: Whiteflies
Diseases: Bacterial wilt, botrytis blight, root rot

HARVESTING

When to harvest: Pick individual leaves anytime after a plant reaches 5 to 6 inches tall. Harvest quantities of leaves for drying anytime in the growing season, picking in the morning when the dew has dried. For maximum fragrance, harvest leaves before flowers appear. Snip off flower clusters when three-quarters of the blooms have opened.
How to harvest: Snip individual leaves and flower

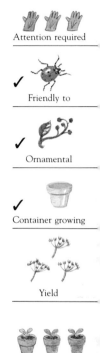

Attention required

Friendly to

Ornamental

Container growing

Yield

Easy to grow

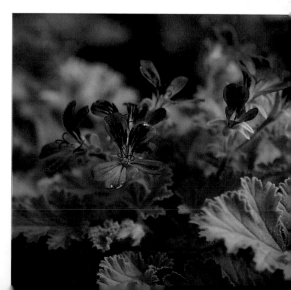

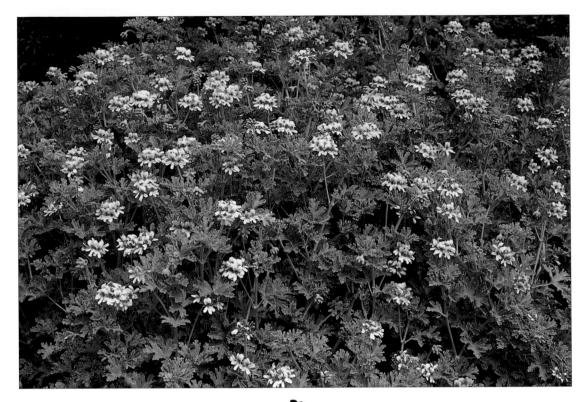

▲ **Beneficial insects** *enjoy the flowers of scented geraniums just as much as people enjoy their wonderfully fragrant foliage.*

clusters where they join the branch, or strip leaves from cut stems.

Drying: Dry leaves and flowers on a screen.

USES

Cooking: Add fresh leaves to jams and jellies, baked goods, and cold sweet drinks and iced tea.

Crafts: Add dried leaves and flowers to potpourris for fragrance and visual appeal.

CULTIVARS AND RELATIVES

It's impossible to go wrong with a scented geranium: They are all wonderful. Connoisseurs collect them by the dozens. A small sampling includes:

- Lemon-scented (*P. crispum* 'Minor'): Tiny leaves on a stiff, upright plant; pinkish flowers.
- Peppermint-scented (*P. tomentosum*): Large velvety leaves; white flowers.
- Rose-scented (*P. graveolens, P. × asperum*): Deeply cut, wrinkly leaves; pink flowers.

TIPS

Growing scented geraniums is like eating potato chips – it's hard to stop at just one. Check mail-order catalogs (see "Resources" on page 155 for sources of scented geraniums) and nearby garden centers to fill out your collection. Because they are so cold-sensitive, many people grow scented geraniums in containers throughout the year. But they add wonderful texture when planted in the garden for the late spring and summer. To propagate scented geraniums, take cuttings from established plants in spring, summer, or early fall. Dig and pot up plants growing in the garden when colder weather nears, or take cuttings when night temperatures fall to 50°F.

Hyssop

Hyssopus officinalis

You'll love hyssop for its blue spires of bloom, but try snipping just a little onto greasy food: It aids in the digestion of fats while adding a strong minty flavor.

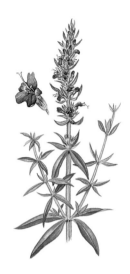

DESCRIPTION
Perennial
1½ to 3 feet tall
Zones 4 to 9
Flowers: Whorls of tiny purple or blue tubular flowers form on tall spikes in midsummer to early fall.
Leaves: Hyssop's slender, pointed leaves are smooth and opposite.
Flavor and fragrance: Hyssop has a strong minty flavor that can become bitter if too much of it is used at one time.

HOW TO GROW
When to plant: Plant seeds a week or two before your last spring frost date. Take cuttings in late spring or early fall and make root divisions in early spring or late summer.
Where to plant: Hyssop prefers full sun but tolerates partial shade.
Soil and fertility: Plant in well-drained sandy soils of moderate fertility. Let the top inch of the soil dry between waterings.

Plant spacing: Space plants 12 inches apart.
Pests: Rarely bothered by pests
Diseases: Susceptible to root rot in soggy soil

HARVESTING
When to harvest: Harvest leaves before the plant flowers, gathering them in the morning when the dew has dried. Pick flowers when the blooms are three-quarters open.
How to harvest: Snip off portions of the stalk when harvesting a small amount of leaves for immediate use and strip the leaves from the stem. Cut whole branches for drying leaves or flowers.
Drying: Hang whole branches upside down to air dry.

USES
Cooking: Use flowers and leaves to give salads a cool, minty flavor. Use flowers and leaves to season stuffing and other poultry dishes, soups, casseroles, and fruit salads.
Teas: Mix hyssop with one of the sweeter mints, such as spearmint, or a more lemony mint like lemon balm.
Arrangements and crafts: Use fresh or dried hyssop flowers in floral arrangements. Dried leaves and flowers add fragrance to potpourris.

◄ **Hyssop** *is especially useful if you keep beehives – its nectar makes a fine honey.*

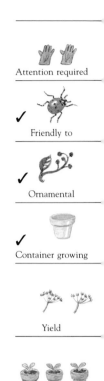

Attention required

✓ Friendly to

✓ Ornamental

✓ Container growing

Yield

Easy to grow

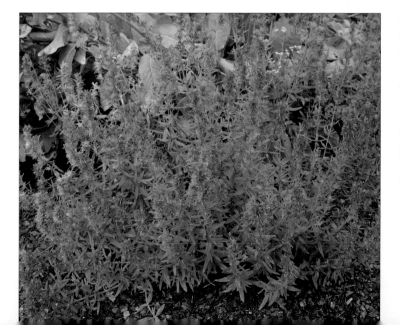

Lavender

Lavandula spp.

Imagine growing so much lavender that you can use it to scent every closet and every drawer and still have lots left to use in winter bouquets and potpourris. This is a beautiful herb to include in any planting.

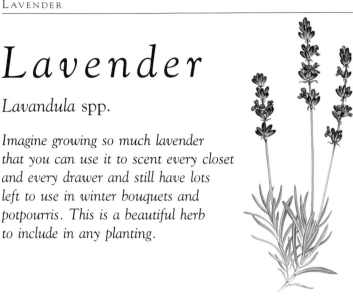

Attention required

 ✓
Friendly to

 ✓
Ornamental

 ✓
Container growing

Yield

Easy to grow

DESCRIPTION
Perennial
To 3 feet tall, depending on species and cultivar
Zones 5 to 8
Flowers: Depending on the species or cultivar, lavender produces slender spikes of blue-purple, lavender, pink, or white flowers in midsummer. Each flower spike may be up to 1 foot long.
Leaves: Lavender's opposite gray-green or silvery green leaves are narrow, smooth-edged, and somewhat hairy.
Flavor and fragrance: Lavender is highly aromatic with a sweet, clean fragrance and flavor with almost-bitter undertones.

HOW TO GROW
When to plant: Start seeds indoors eight to ten weeks before your last spring frost date. Seeds require light for germination. Transplant seedlings to the garden after that date. Take softwood cuttings in late spring.
Where to plant: Lavender

prefers full sun but tolerates partial shade.
Soil and fertility: Plant in well-drained moderately fertile soil. Lavender prefers alkaline soil. Allow the top inch of soil to dry between waterings.
Plant spacing: Space plants 1 to 3 feet apart.
Pests: Largely pest-free
Diseases: Leaf spot can develop in high temperatures and humidity. Plant in raised beds and pick off any infected

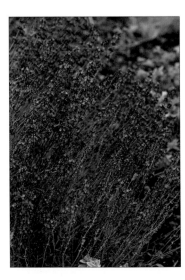

leaves. Prune to improve air circulation around the stems. Plants in consistently moist soil are prone to root rot.

HARVESTING
When to harvest: Harvest flower spikes and stems when flowers are nearly open.
How to harvest: Cut flowers several inches below the bloom. Cut stems to within one node of the woody growth when harvesting for leaves or arrangements.
Drying: To dry lavender for arrangements, lay it on flat screens so the branches dry in an attractive shape. Or hang stems upside down in a hot, well-ventilated location.

USES
Cooking: Add fresh or dried flowers to baked goods and jellies. Mix the flowers with black tea for a fragrant cup.
Medicinal: A strong tea is calming. Cold lavender teas applied to a washcloth make a compress to relieve headaches.
Cosmetic: Use in skin oils, creams, and lotions and in conditioners for oily hair.
Arrangements and crafts: Use lavender flowers and leaves in potpourris and sachets.

◄ **'Munstead' lavender** *produces huge numbers of densely packed, fragrant blossoms.*

Lemon balm

Melissa officinalis

The signature scent of lemon balm will envelop you every time you brush against its leaves. Don't be afraid to plant this mint – it isn't invasive, and you'll use a lot of it.

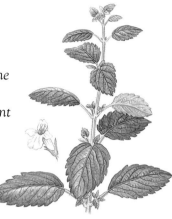

DESCRIPTION

Perennial
1 to 2 feet tall
Zones 4 to 9
Flowers: Clusters of ½-inch-long tubular whitish flowers bloom in midsummer where the leaves join the stems.
Leaves: The opposite leaves are bright green and have toothed edges. Plants die back over winter.
Flavor and fragrance: Lemon balm has a honey-sweet lemon flavor and fragrance.

HOW TO GROW

When to plant: Sow seeds in the garden about two weeks before your last spring frost date. Or start seeds indoors about eight weeks before your last spring frost date and transplant seedlings to the garden a week before that date. Divide plants in spring or early summer; replant and water well until they are established.
Where to plant: Lemon balm prefers full sun in the North, filtered shade in the South.
Soil and fertility: Plant in well-drained soil of average fertility.
Plant spacing: Space plants 1½ to 2 feet apart.
Pests: Usually pest-free
Diseases: Powdery mildew may appear late in the season.

HARVESTING

When to harvest: Harvest leaves anytime for immediate

◄ **Golden lemon balm's** *"quilted" leaves add an appealing accent to fresh bouquets.*

use, gathering them in the morning after the dew has dried. Collect leaves for drying before the plant flowers.
How to harvest: Snip off stem tips when harvesting only a small amount of leaves. For drying in quantity, cut whole stems, 4 inches above the soil surface.
Drying: Lemon balm tends to darken when air dried. Strip leaves from stems and place them on the fruit leather insert of a dehydrator.
Freezing: Freeze whole lemon balm leaves in ice cubes for a decorative effect in iced teas.

USES

Cooking: Use minced fresh lemon balm in salads, sauces, sauerkraut, and stuffing, and sprinkle over vegetables, chicken, and fish dishes.
Teas: Lemon balm is an excellent tea herb, either alone or in combination with other herbs.
Cosmetic: Use lemon balm to condition oily hair.
Crafts: Mix dried leaves in potpourris.

TIPS

Lemon balm is not as invasive as many other herbs in the mint family, but it does self-sow abundantly. Seedlings are easy to weed out, or simply snip off flowering stalks before they set seed.

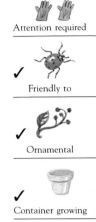

Attention required

✓ Friendly to

✓ Ornamental

✓ Container growing

Yield

Easy to grow

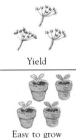

Lemongrass

Cymbopogon citratus

Expand your cooking repertoire with Asian dishes that come to life with the authentic flavor of lemongrass. Or simply add this herb to teas or sauces for its fresh, lemony taste.

Attention required

Friendly to ✗

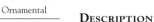
Ornamental ✗

Container growing ✓

Yield

Easy to grow

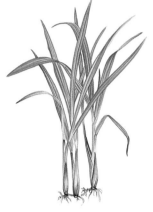

DESCRIPTION
Perennial, grown in containers in cooler zones
3 to 5 feet tall; up to 4 feet wide
Zones 9 to 10
Flowers: Lemongrass rarely flowers, but when it does, the inconspicuous greenish flowers form at the top of stalks.
Leaves: The straplike leaves grow in a grassy clump. The base of each leaf is enlarged and whitish colored. North of Zone 9, overwinter indoors.
Flavor and fragrance: Lemongrass has a sharp lemon flavor and fragrance.

HOW TO GROW
When to plant: Start seeds in pots or seedling flats in early spring. Transplant after all danger of frost is past. Divide roots by digging entire plant and dividing it into two or three pieces. Replant at the same depth as before. Divide established plants in spring and early summer. When dividing lemongrass, snip off all but 3 to 4 inches of the leaves to reduce

the amount of water lost through leaves.
Where to plant: Lemongrass prefers full sun.
Soil and fertility: Plant in rich, moist garden soil. In containers, use a medium containing one-third compost, one-third good topsoil, one-sixth peat moss, and one-sixth vermiculite. Feed container plants with liquid fish emulsion and seaweed at monthly intervals during the summer.
Plant spacing: Space garden plants 2 to 4 feet apart. For container plants, start seeds in a 6-inch pot and move into successively larger pots as the clump grows. A mature clump of lemongrass grows best in a 5-gallon nursery pot.
Pests: Lemongrass is not bothered by pests other than cats, which eat the leaves and may dig up the plant.
Diseases: Largely disease-free

HARVESTING
When to harvest: Harvest leaves and stems anytime, once the plants are a foot tall.

How to harvest: Gently pull off older outside bulbous stems from base for use in cooking. The young leaves can also be cut off and used. Snip off leaves for tea making.
Drying: In dehydrator.
Freezing: In light oil or water ice cubes.

USES
Cooking: Use the leaves fresh, dried, or frozen, and bulbous stems in Thai and Vietnamese dishes, stir-fries, soups, pasta, tofu, and vegetables.
Teas: Use leaves in mixed herbal teas.
Crafts: Lemongrass leaves add a lemony fragrance to potpourris and sachets.

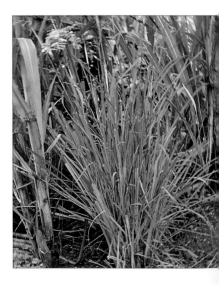

▲ **Lemongrass** *looks a bit weedy, but its flavor makes it an herb worth growing.*

Lemon verbena

Aloysia triphylla

Lemon verbena is one of those herbs you'll never want to be without. Hang a basket where you can rub a leaf when you pass – you'll never need or want another room freshener!

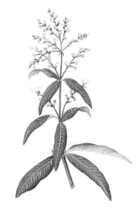

DESCRIPTION

Perennial, grown in containers in cooler zones
To 2 feet tall and wide
Zones 9 and 10
Flowers: In late summer to early fall, spikes of tiny, tubular, lavender-colored flowers grow where the leaves join the stems.
Leaves: The narrow pointed leaves grow in whorls of three or four. Some plants have slightly hairy leaves. The stems become woody with age.
Flavor and fragrance: Lemon verbena has a complex lemon flavor and fragrance with undertones of sweetness.

HOW TO GROW

When to plant: North of Zone 9, grow lemon verbena in containers. Seeds are hard to find and difficult to germinate, so it's best to buy a plant. To propagate, take softwood cuttings in late spring or early summer. Cuttings can be a challenge, too; make a tent of plastic over the flat to keep humidity high.
Where to plant: Lemon verbena prefers full sun. During the winter, keep indoor plants in a south window or under plant lights.
Soil and fertility: Plant in fertile soil. Pot up in humus-rich soil, and fertilize with liquid seaweed and fish emulsion every month during the summer. In fall, cut the plant back by about half and repot in new soil. Do not fertilize during the winter.
Plant spacing: Space outdoor plants 12 inches apart. Potted plants need a 10- to 12-inch container.
Pests: Spider mites, whiteflies
Diseases: Usually disease-free

HARVESTING

When to harvest: Harvest leaves and stems anytime after the plant reaches 8 inches tall.
How to harvest: Snip off branch tips. Cut whole stems for drying larger quantities; cut the entire plant back to about 2 inches above the ground in midsummer to promote growth.
Drying: Dry on screens or in a dehydrator.

USES

Cooking: Add the lemon-flavored leaves to sauces, marinades, and salad dressings. Use the fresh leaves to add lemony flavor to fruit salads, desserts, and beverages.
Teas: Lemon verbena makes a good tea alone or in combination with other herbs.
Oils: Combine with light oils such as safflower or canola.
Cosmetic: Lemon verbena adds a pleasant fragrance to hand lotions.
Crafts: Add to potpourris and sachets for fragrance.

TIPS

Place pots of lemon verbena around the dining area so people can add leaves to their iced drinks.

▼ **Lemon verbena** *plants remain healthy and productive for years when given good care.*

Attention required

✓ Friendly to

✓ Ornamental

✓ Container growing

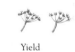
Yield

Easy to grow

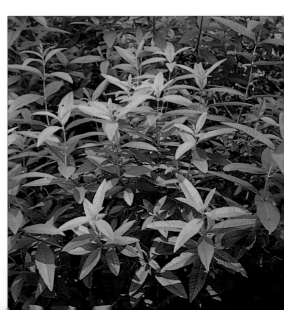

Lovage

Levisticum officinale

Tall, shapely lovage plants at the back of the garden give it a lush appearance. Just one plant will supply your needs for a year, but you may want more for their ornamental value.

Attention required

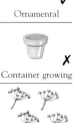

✓

Friendly to

✓

Ornamental

✗

Container growing

Yield

Easy to grow

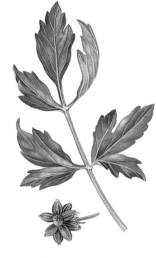

DESCRIPTION
Perennial
6 feet tall; 2 to 3 feet wide
Zones 4 to 8
Flowers: Umbels of tiny yellowish white flowers appear in mid- to late summer.
Leaves: Glossy, compound, celerylike leaves grow from thick stalks. Plants die back in the winter.
Flavor and fragrance: Lovage's flavor and fragrance strongly resemble that of celery.

▼ **Lovage** *leaves lend a splash of bright green and an upright form to fresh arrangements.*

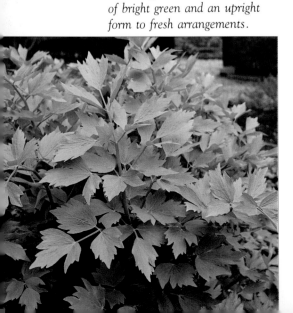

HOW TO GROW
When to plant: Lovage seeds must be fresh to germinate. Gather seeds from a plant in the neighborhood or purchase them in late summer and plant immediately. Or buy plants (you'll only need one or two) from a nursery and plant them in the garden just before your last spring frost date or in late summer. Divide mature plants in spring to early summer.
Where to plant: Lovage prefers partial or filtered shade but will tolerate full shade.
Soil and fertility: Plant in well-drained moist soil with good fertility. Mulch with ½ inch of compost in spring.
Plant spacing: Allow 2 square feet per plant.
Pests: Leafminers cause clear or whitish tunneling marks in the leaves. In most cases, only a few leaves will be affected and the plant won't be harmed. If the infestation becomes severe, pick off and destroy any affected leaves.
Diseases: Rarely bothered by diseases.

HARVESTING
When to harvest: Harvest leaves anytime during the growing season for immediate use. For the best quality, gather them in the morning after the dew has dried. Harvest leaves for drying before the plant flowers. Harvest entire ripe seed heads in late summer.
How to harvest: Snip off leaves as needed. If harvesting for drying, cut 1- to 3-foot sections of the stems. Enclose seed heads as they begin to ripen.
Drying: Lovage loses flavor unless it dries quickly. Use a dehydrator.
Freezing: Blanch leaves before freezing in ice cubes or oil.

USES
Cooking: Use celery-flavored lovage leaves, fresh, frozen, or dried, anywhere you would use celery, particularly in cheese and egg dishes and soups and stews. Include the fresh leaves in salads. Lovage stems are very fibrous; if you use them in cooking, remove them before serving.
Medicinal: Apply a strong infusion of lovage to wounds as an antiseptic. Lovage tea stimulates digestion.

TIPS
Even if you never snip a leaf off the plant, you'll love lovage for its impressive height. Plant it toward the rear of a partially shaded area.

Marjoram, sweet

Origanum majorana

Sweet marjoram smells so good you can use it to add fragrance to potpourris and sachets for the linen closet. But save some to eat, too – it's a sweeter version of oregano.

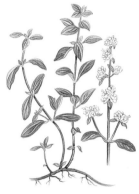

DESCRIPTION

Perennial grown as annual
1 foot tall
Zones 9 to 10
Flowers: In late summer to early fall, clustered flower spikes appear. The flower buds look like knots before they open into tiny white or pink blooms.
Leaves: Sweet marjoram has opposite, fuzzy, oval leaves, from ¼ to 1 inch long.
Flavor and fragrance: Sweet marjoram has a flavor that is both sweet and spicy and a delicate aroma.

HOW TO GROW

When to plant: Start seeds indoors about eight to ten weeks before your last spring frost date, planting three to five seeds in each pot. Sweet marjoram is slow to germinate and tiny when young. Transplant seedlings to the garden after all danger of frost has passed. Take cuttings in spring or early summer.
Where to plant: Sweet marjoram prefers full sun but tolerates partial shade.

Soil and fertility: Plant in sandy, well-drained soil of low to moderate fertility. Allow the top inch of soil to dry between waterings.
Plant spacing: Space plants 6 to 8 inches apart.
Pests: Usually pest-free
Diseases: Usually disease-free

HARVESTING

When to harvest: Pick individual leaves anytime after the plant is 6 to 8 inches tall. For best quality, gather leaves in the morning after the dew dries. Cut stems with leaves before plants bloom for drying in quantity.
How to harvest: Snip branch tips when taking just a bit. Cut whole stems for drying.

▶ **Sweet marjoram** *combines well with other herbs in the garden.*

Drying: Hang stems upside down to air dry.
Freezing: Freeze leaves in oils, butter, or ice cubes.

USES

Cooking: Use fresh leaves in salads or for garnishes. Sweet marjoram is somewhat milder and sweeter than oregano but carries much of the same flavor. Use fresh, frozen, or dried leaves wherever you would use oregano. Use it to season cheese, beef, pork, and cabbage-family vegetables.
Medicinal: Sweet marjoram infusions settle upset stomachs and are used as a gargle for mouth and throat inflammations.
Cosmetic: Add to bathwater for wonderful fragrance and energizing effect.
Crafts: Add to sachets or a potpourri mix.

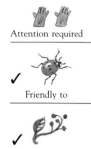
Attention required

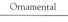
Friendly to

Ornamental

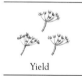
Container growing

Yield

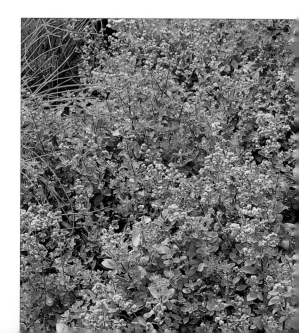
Easy to grow

Mints

Mentha spp.

Indulge yourself with mints by buying small pots of several different kinds. These plants spread so easily it won't be long before you have a sizable mint garden filled with a variety of flavors.

Attention required

 ✓

Friendly to

✓

Ornamental

✓

Container growing

Yield

Easy to grow

DESCRIPTION

Perennial

To 2 feet tall, depending on species and cultivar

Zones 5 to 9

Flowers: Spikes of tiny purple, pink, or white flowers bloom above the leaves in mid- to late summer.

Leaves: Opposite leaves in many shades of green, most with toothed edges, cover characteristic square stems.

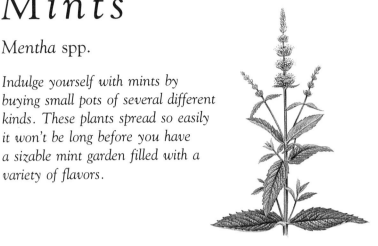

▼ **Mints** *grow vigorously in most gardens.*

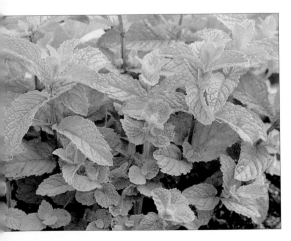

Plants die back over the winter.

Flavor and fragrance: Mints vary a great deal in flavor and fragrance. For example, spearmint and apple mint are sweetish, while peppermint is cooling and has a sharper flavor.

HOW TO GROW

When to plant: Few mints come true from seed. You can transplant purchased plants into your garden anytime from early spring through summer. If you want to try mints from seed, start them indoors eight to ten weeks before your last spring frost date and transplant them to the garden a week or two before that date. Take cuttings from established plants before they bloom. Divide plants in early spring or, in southern locations, in late summer or early fall.

Where to plant: Mints prefer partial or filtered shade but tolerate both full sun and shade.

Soil and fertility: Mints grow best in moist soils of moderate fertility. High fertility levels make them more susceptible to diseases such as rust. In average soil, apply no more than ½ inch of compost in alternate years. Plants tolerate high humidity.

Plant spacing: Start plants 18 to 24 inches apart; they spread very fast. Unless you want a huge mint patch, sink barriers 12 inches into the soil on all sides of the plant to prevent its taking over the garden. Or grow mints in 5-gallon buckets with drainage holes, buried in the ground. Mints also grow well in large containers.

Pests: Aphids, spider mites, mint flea beetles, cutworms

Diseases: Rust, verticillium wilt, anthracnose

HARVESTING

When to harvest: Gather leaves from mint anytime after a plant reaches 6 to 8 inches tall. Gather leafy stems in the morning after the dew dries. For drying, pick before or after the plant has bloomed.

How to harvest: Snip off the tips of branches. For drying, cut stems 4 to 6 inches above the soil surface during the early summer, and make a second cutting 1 inch above the soil surface in fall.

Drying: Hang leafy stems upside down to air dry or dry them in a dehydrator. Peppermint holds its fragrance and flavor better than other mints when dried.

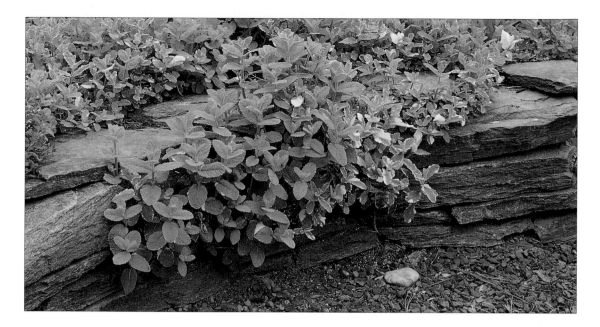

Freezing: Freeze leaves in butter, oils, or ice cubes.

USES

Cooking: Mints complement the flavors of meat, fish, and vegetable dishes. Use fresh leaves in salads, and add fresh or dried leaves to lamb stews, dried beans, or cooked grains. Mints heighten the flavor of fresh peas, steamed new potatoes, or carrots. They add zip to cream sauces and make wonderful jellies. Experiment and you'll find hundreds of ways to use mint in your cooking.

Teas: Mints make delicious teas. Try mixing different mints, or add some mint to your other tea herbs.

Medicinal: A strong infusion of mint settles the stomach and relieves flatulence. Spearmint and peppermint infusions, alone or with chamomile, promote sleep.

Cosmetic: Splash a refreshing infusion of mint over your face on a hot summer day; add mint to a conditioner for oily hair.

Crafts: Add fragrant mint leaves to potpourris and sachets.

▲ **Variegated mint** *offers beauty and fragrance.*

TIPS

Rodents dislike fresh mint.

CULTIVARS AND RELATIVES

- Apple mint (M. *suaveolens*): Very sturdy plant with gray-green foliage and a slight apple scent.
- Corsican mint (M. *requienii*): Small-leaved plant excellent for using as a fine-textured groundcover or between paving stones; Zones 6 to 10.
- Ginger mint (M. × *gentilis* 'Variegata'): Highly ornamental variegated leaves that taste like mint with a hint of ginger.
- Lemon mint (M. × *piperita* var. *citrata*): Leaves carry a fresh, lemony scent; also called orange mint, eau-de-cologne mint, and bergamot mint.
- Peppermint (M. × *piperita*): Features the familiar strong aroma most people associate with mint and a slightly spicy flavor.
- Pineapple mint (M. *suaveolens* 'Variegata'): Lovely variegated leaves have a fruity scent slightly reminiscent of apple, not pineapple.
- Spearmint (M. *spicata*): Another familiar mint with a sweeter, more fruity taste than peppermint.

Nasturtium

Tropaeolum majus

Fill a sunny window box with colorful nasturtiums – you'll have a lovely ornamental planting that provides you with a steady supply of spicy salad garnishes near at hand.

Attention required

 ✓
Friendly to

 ✓
Ornamental

 ✓
Container growing

Yield

Easy to grow

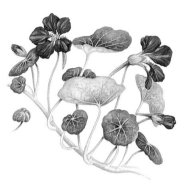

DESCRIPTION
Annual
To 1 foot tall; vining to 6 feet
Flowers: Cheery, open, funnel-shaped flowers bloom from summer through fall in colors from cream to brilliant reds, oranges, and yellows. Each five-petaled flower is about 1½ to 2 inches across and has a long spur at the base.
Leaves: Nasturtium's round, long-stemmed leaves feature wavy or slightly lobed margins. The size of the leaves depends on how rich your soil is. In poor soils, they grow only 1 to 2 inches across; in ideal conditions, about 3 to 4 inches; and in soils that are too rich, as large as 6 inches across.

Flavor and fragrance: Nasturtium leaves and flowers taste spicy and almost peppery with no noticeable fragrance.

HOW TO GROW
When to plant: Sow seeds in the garden around the time of your last spring frost date. Or start them indoors, in plantable pots of peat or newspaper, four to five weeks before your last spring frost. Transplant after all chance of frost has passed.
Where to plant: Nasturtiums prefer full sun. Plants will survive in filtered shade but do not flower as well.
Soil and fertility: Plant in well-drained, only moderately fertile soil.

Plant spacing: Space plants 12 inches apart.
Pests: Aphids, leafminers
Diseases: Bacterial wilt, leaf spot, verticillium wilt

HARVESTING
When to harvest: You can pick leaves as soon as the plant is 6 inches tall. Pick flowers just as they open. Collect the green seedpods when they are just over ¼ inch in diameter.
How to harvest: Cut leaves and flowers with their stems attached. Remove old flowers to prolong the bloom period. To collect seeds, stop deadheading in mid-August.
Preserving seeds: Place fresh green seedpods in a heat-proof jar and pour heated vinegar over them. Let them cure for a week before using. Store in the refrigerator.

USES
Cooking: Use both leaves and flowers in fresh salads or as a garnish. Use preserved seedpods as a substitute for capers in tartar sauces and spiced mayonnaises.
Cosmetic: To clear skin eruptions, crush the seeds very finely and spread them on a hot washcloth. Hold the cloth against the skin until it cools.

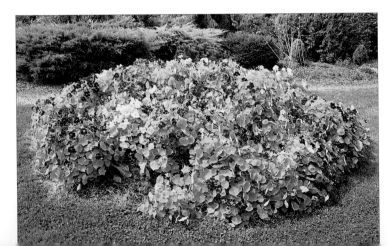

◄ **Nasturtiums** *produce more flowers when grown in soil of only average fertility.*

Oregano

Origanum vulgare

Today we think of pizza and spaghetti sauce when we think of oregano, but culinary uses were once secondary to its medicinal qualities. Oregano tea clears the nasal passages and eases the sore throat of the common cold.

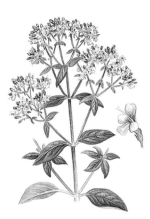

DESCRIPTION

Perennial
2 feet tall
Zones 5 to 9
Flowers: Culinary oregano bears spikes of tiny white flowers above the leaves in midsummer.
Leaves: Carried on square stems, oregano leaves are opposite, with toothed or smooth edges, and range from ½ inch to 2 inches long.
Flavor and fragrance: Oregano has a spicy, pungent flavor with an undertone of sweetness; it is highly aromatic.

HOW TO GROW

When to plant: Buy plants to be sure of getting the flavor you want. If you want to try growing oregano from seed, sow three to five seeds indoors in individual pots eight weeks before your last spring frost date. Transplant seedlings to the garden a week before that date. Propagate by layering: Bend stems to the ground and cover them with soil in early summer; transplant the newly rooted plants in early fall. Take cuttings in late spring, before bloom.
Where to plant: Oregano prefers full sun.
Soil and fertility: Plant in well-drained soils of average fertility. Allow the top inch of soil to dry out between waterings.
Plant spacing: Allow 1 foot between groups of plants.
Pests: Aphids, leafminers, spider mites
Diseases: Root rot, leaf spot

HARVESTING

When to harvest: Cut small sprigs anytime after the plant reaches 6 inches tall. Harvest whole stems for drying just before bloom. Cut the entire plant back to 2 to 3 inches above ground in August to promote new growth.
How to harvest: Snip off the ends of the stems with sharp scissors. For drying, cut off whole stems an inch or two above the soil surface.
Drying: Hang leafy stems upside down to air dry. Or strip leaves from stems and dry the leaves on the fruit leather insert in a dehydrator.

USES

Cooking: Tomato sauce isn't tomato sauce without oregano. Use the leaves, fresh or dried, to season cheeses, eggs, most vegetables, and meats.
Oils: Add oregano to olive oil to create a perfect seasoning for Italian dishes.
Arrangements and crafts: Add fresh or dried flower spikes to arrangements.

TIPS

Plant Greek oregano (*O. heracleoticum*, also sold as *O. vulgare* subsp. *hirtum*) for culinary use.

Attention required

✓ Friendly to

✓ Ornamental

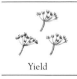
✓ Container growing

Yield

Easy to grow

▼ **Golden oregano** *sparkles amid the rocks.*

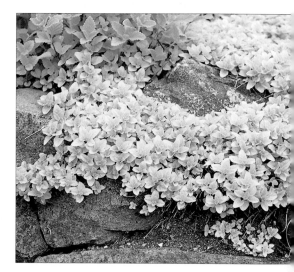

Parsley

Petroselinum crispum

Don't limit parsley's uses to garnishing other foods – this herb is so versatile that you can add it to almost any dish. Chewing a sprig after you eat cleans and freshens the breath.

Attention required

 ✗

Friendly to

 ✓

Ornamental

 ✓

Container growing

Yield

Easy to grow

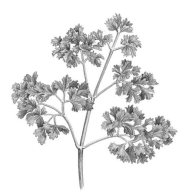

DESCRIPTION

Biennial, usually grown as an annual
8 to 12 inches tall
Zones 5 to 9
Flowers: Flat Queen-Anne's-lace-like umbels of tiny greenish yellow flowers bloom in late spring of the second year of growth.
Leaves: Curly parsley has fine, ferny, curled and ruffled, deep green leaves that are held on long stems from the crown of the plant. The foliage of flat-leaved types resembles that of celery.
Flavor and fragrance: Parsley has a fresh, tangy flavor with an undertone of sweetness. Its fragrance is much like its flavor.

HOW TO GROW

When to plant: Parsley seed is notorious for being slow to germinate. Start with plants, or try the seed pretreatment described in "Tips." Sow seeds indoors in peat or newspaper pots eight to ten weeks before your last spring frost date. Transplant seedlings to the

garden one week before that date. Transplant carefully – injury to the taproot can cause plants to flower and set seed prematurely.
Where to plant: Prefers full sun or filtered shade; tolerates shade.
Soil and fertility: Plant parsley in well-drained moist soil of high fertility.
Plant spacing: Space plants 10 to 12 inches apart.
Pests: Parsleyworms (swallowtail butterfly caterpillars), aphids, carrot weevils
Diseases: Crown rot

HARVESTING

When to harvest: Harvest leaves anytime after plant has grown at least eight leaves.
How to harvest: Cut off stems and leaves 1 inch above the crown of the plant.
Freezing: Freeze leaves on a baking sheet, then store them in freezer containers.
Drying: Dry parsley in a dehydrator for the best flavor and color retention.

USES

Cooking: Add fresh, frozen, or dried leaves to soups, stews, casseroles, vegetable dishes, and fish and poultry. Use fresh leaves in salads or as a garnish.
Cosmetic: In hair conditioners, parsley helps prevent dandruff and conditions dry hair.

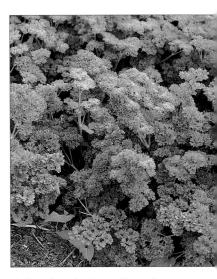

▲ **Parsley** *feeds swallowtail butterflies, too!*

TIPS

Parsley seed is coated with a compound that inhibits germination. Overcome this by soaking the seed overnight and then pouring it into a fine-mesh strainer. During the next two to three days, frequently pour cool water over it. At night, keep the seeds in a glass jar with a bit of water in it so they don't dry out.

Pennyroyal

Mentha pulegium, English pennyroyal
Hedeoma pulegioides, American pennyroyal

Pennyroyal comes into its own when you need to repel pesky insects. Rub it on yourself at picnics or when you're gardening during "buggy" times.

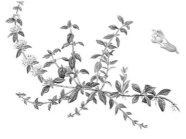

DESCRIPTION

English pennyroyal
Perennial
To 1 foot tall
Zones 5 to 9

American pennyroyal
Annual
12 to 15 inches tall

Flowers: Tubular, ¼-inch-long, lavender blue flowers bloom in mid- to late summer in whorls where the leaves join the stems.
Leaves: Both pennyroyals are members of the mint family and have characteristic square stems. English pennyroyal forms a low carpet of opposite, ½-inch-long, slightly hairy leaves on prostrate stems. American pennyroyal is a more upright plant with leaves up to 1 inch long. In protected locations, English pennyroyal is evergreen in winter.
Flavor and fragrance: Pennyroyal has a minty fragrance. Do not eat it.

HOW TO GROW

When to plant: Sow seeds directly in the garden about two weeks before your last spring frost date. Take cuttings or layer English pennyroyal in early summer; divide plants in spring or fall.
Where to plant: Prefers full sun to partial shade.
Soil and fertility: English pennyroyal prefers moist soil with average fertility; apply compost in alternate years. American pennyroyal requires a fertile, well-drained site; allow the top inch of soil to dry between waterings.
Plant spacing: Allow 6 inches between English plants, and 8 to 10 inches between American plants.
Pests: Aphids, spider mites, mint flea beetles, cutworms
Diseases: Rust, verticillium wilt, anthracnose

HARVESTING

When to harvest: Harvest individual sprigs in the morning after the plant is at least 8 inches tall or the stems are 8 inches long. For drying, harvest in spring and summer before and after bloom.

How to harvest: Snip off stem tips or cut whole stems, several inches above the surface of the soil or the crown of the plant.
Drying: Hang upside down to air dry.

USES

Insect repellent: Rub pennyroyal on your skin to repel insects. Or pick an insect-chasing bouquet for the picnic table, and crush the leaves occasionally to release their fragrance. Add dried pennyroyal leaves to a flea-repellent cushion for pets.

TIPS

Do not take internally; pennyroyal is a strong poison.

Attention required

✓

Friendly to

✓

Ornamental

✓

Container growing

Yield

Easy to grow

▼ **English pennyroyal** *is almost indestructible.*

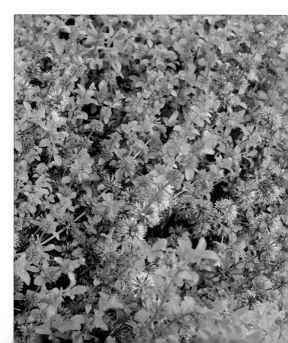

Rosemary

Rosmarinus officinalis

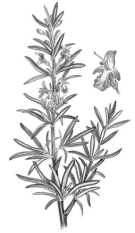

Greek students once wore garlands of rosemary in their hair while taking examinations because they believed it strengthened the memory. Though a wreath may have no effect on your mind power, the flavor of this herb is indispensable in the kitchen.

Attention required

 ✓

Friendly to

 ✓

Ornamental

 ✓

Container growing

Yield

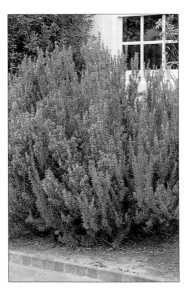

Easy to grow

DESCRIPTION

Perennial, grown in containers in cooler zones
2 to 6 feet tall
Zones 8 to 10
Flowers: Tiny pink to purple flowers bloom in clusters of two or three along the branches in late winter to early spring.
Leaves: Rosemary's needlelike leathery leaves are ⅓ to 1½ inches long, opposite, and evergreen.
Flavor and fragrance: Rosemary has a strong, pungent flavor and aroma with a hint of pine.

HOW TO GROW

When to plant: Rosemary seeds grow so slowly that it's preferable to buy plants. In warm climates, plant outdoors anytime. North of Zone 8, keep plants indoors until night temperatures are at least 55°F. Take cuttings in late summer and layer plants in early summer.
Where to plant: Prefers full sun during the growing season. To overwinter indoors, place in a south or southeast window.

Soil and fertility: Plant rosemary in extremely well-drained soil. Allow the top 1 to 1½ inches of the soil surface to dry between waterings. Apply ½ inch of compost around plants every other year.
Plant spacing: Allow 1 to 3 feet between plants outdoors. Container-grown plants require deep pots. As your plant grows, transplant it into larger pots. Mature plants may require a 10-gallon pot.
Pests: Scale, mealybugs, spider mites, whiteflies
Diseases: Root rot, botrytis blight

HARVESTING

When to harvest: Harvest stems and leaves anytime.
How to harvest: Snip branch tips when you need only a small amount. To harvest larger quantities, cut stems back to within one or two leaf nodes above woody growth.
Drying: Dry flat on screens or in a dehydrator.
Freezing: Freeze whole sprigs of rosemary.

USES

Cooking: Use fresh or dried leaves of rosemary with pork, lamb, poultry, fish, tofu, eggs, cheese, breads, stuffings, and many vegetables.
Oils: Flavor olive oil or lighter oils such as safflower or canola with a few sprigs of rosemary.
Cosmetic: Add rosemary to your bathwater for a stimulating effect. Use it in hair rinses and conditioners to add highlights to dark hair, to condition oily hair, to help prevent dandruff, and to give hair body.
Crafts: Add its fragrance to potpourris and sachets.

▼ **Rosemary** *makes a fragrant foundation planting for homes in Zones 8 to 10.*

Rue

Ruta graveolens

The unusual blue-green color and soft texture of rue make it a striking accent plant. Even if you never harvest it, you'll enjoy it in a perennial border where its foliage can set off silvers, whites, and purples.

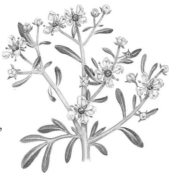

DESCRIPTION

Perennial
To 3 feet tall
Zones 4 to 9
Flowers: Clusters of yellow to yellow-green ½-inch flowers bloom at the top of the plant in midsummer.
Leaves: Rue's evergreen foliage is an attractive blue-green color. The alternate 3- to 5-inch-long leaves consist of smaller, rounded leaflets that are sometimes covered with a whitish powder.
Flavor and fragrance: Rue is not recommended for internal use; it has a strong, bitter aroma.

HOW TO GROW

When to plant: Rue seedlings grow slowly, so you may want to buy a plant instead. Start seeds indoors at least eight weeks before your last spring frost date. Wait until the seedlings reach 2 to 3 inches tall before transplanting them to the garden in late spring. Take cuttings or layer plants in spring and early summer.

Where to plant: Rue prefers full sun but tolerates partial shade.
Soil and fertility: Plant in well-drained soil of low to moderate fertility.
Plant spacing: Space plants 1½ to 2 feet apart.
Pests: Pest-free
Diseases: Susceptible to root rot in poorly drained soils or when overwatered

HARVESTING

When to harvest: Harvest stems with leaves before the plant flowers. For best quality, gather leafy stems in the morning after the dew dries. Harvest seedpods for dried arrangements in late summer when they are fully grown but not yet brown. For best success in drying seedpods, gather them in dry weather.
How to harvest: Cut at the base of leaf stems. See "Tips" below for harvesting precautions.
Drying: Hang stems upside down to air dry.

USES

Arrangements: Use dried stems of leaves and seedpods in dried arrangements.
Insect repellent: Include dried leaves of rue in pest-repelling cushions for your pet.

TIPS

Many people are sensitive to the oil contained in the leaves of rue and develop dermatitis ranging from small blisters to a severely painful rash if they come into contact with it. To be on the safe side, wear gloves and long sleeves when working with the plant. Rue is said to interfere with the growth of many plants, particularly cabbage-family crops, sage, and basil. Plant rue at least 10 feet away from any of these plants.

Attention required

✗ Friendly to

✓ Ornamental

✗ Container growing

Yield

Easy to grow

▼ **Rue** *is a difficult companion for many other plants, so choose a spot for it with care.*

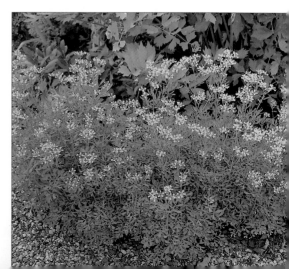

Saffron crocus

Crocus sativus

Attention required

✓

Friendly to

✓

Ornamental

❌

Container growing

Yield

Easy to grow

Plant some saffron crocus in the front of your chrysanthemum beds to brighten up the fall garden. If you pluck the saffron threads to use in cooking, you'll be getting double pleasure from this plant.

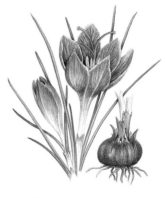

DESCRIPTION
Perennial
1 foot tall
Zones 6 to 9
Flowers: Lovely lavender, white, or purplish flowers bloom in fall. They look just like the crocuses that bloom in the spring garden. The flowers have vivid orange-yellow stigmas.
Leaves: Narrow grasslike leaves, 6 to 12 inches long, appear in spring and die back once hot weather sets in.
Flavor and fragrance: Saffron is highly flavorful and aromatic with a spicy, pungent, and slightly bitter taste.

HOW TO GROW
When to plant: Plant saffron corms in spring or fall, placing them root side down, 3 to 4 inches below the soil surface. Lift and divide the corms every three to four years in early summer after the foliage dies back; replant immediately.
Where to plant: Saffron prefers partial shade but tolerates full sun.
Soil and fertility: Plant in well-drained soil of average fertility.
Plant spacing: Leave about 6 inches between corms. Plants will produce baby corms that eventually fill in the group.

Pests: Pest-free
Diseases: Susceptible to root rot in soggy soil conditions

HARVESTING
When to harvest: Harvest the orange-yellow stigmas in fall when the flowers are fully open. Gather them in the morning just after the flowers open and before pollinating insects begin visiting the blossoms.
How to harvest: With tweezers, pull out the three stigmas in each flower.
Drying: Dry the stigmas on the fruit leather insert of your dehydrator, or place them between sheets of brown paper in an airy location.

USES
Cooking: Saffron threads (stigmas) are used in many rice dishes as well as with vegetables, meats, seafood, poultry, and in baked goods. They add a sharp, almost medicinal flavor, and a beautiful orange-yellow color.

TIPS
Only *C. sativus* produces saffron threads. Each flower produces only three stigmas. About 100,000 plants are required to produce a pound of threads. It takes about six plants to grow the quantity of saffron called for in most recipes. But the flowers are a pretty addition to the fall garden, even if you only season a single recipe.

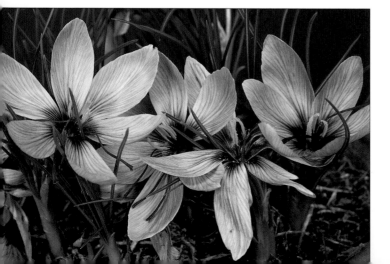

◀ **Saffron crocus** *looks like any other flowering bulb. Who would guess it yields saffron threads?*

Sage

Salvia officinalis

Sage has a warm, homey aroma that instantly gives a feeling of comfort. Let its fragrance drift through your kitchen by crushing a few leaves and boiling them in a small open saucepan.

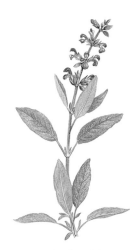

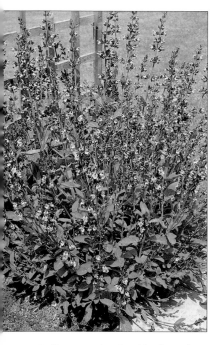

▲ **Sage** *retains its tidy form for about three years.*

DESCRIPTION

Perennial
2½ to 3 feet tall
Zones 4 to 8
Flowers: Sage's small tubular pink, purple, blue, or white flowers grow in whorls of four to eight at points where the leaves attach to the stems. Most cultivars bloom in late spring to early summer.
Leaves: The 2-inch-long gray-green leaves may be hairy, velvety, or pebbly looking, depending on the cultivar. The stems become woody as a plant ages.
Flavor and fragrance: Sage has a warm, pungent flavor with a hint of camphor. Its aroma echoes its flavor.

HOW TO GROW

When to plant: Freeze seeds for at least three days before planting. Cover seeds thoroughly when you plant them; sage germinates best in darkness. Sow seeds indoors about eight weeks before your last spring frost date; transplant seedlings to the garden a week before that date. Or plant prefrozen seeds in the garden one to two weeks before your last spring frost date. Take cuttings or make root divisions in early summer.

Where to plant: Prefers full sun.
Soil and fertility: Plant sage in well-drained soil of average fertility. Apply ½ inch of compost in the second and third years of growth.
Plant spacing: Space plants 2 feet apart.
Pests: Spider mites, spittlebugs, slugs
Diseases: Bacterial wilt, root rot, verticillium wilt

HARVESTING

When to harvest: Pick individual leaves anytime. Harvest quantities of leaves for drying in mid- to late summer.
How to harvest: Snip off individual leaves. Cut whole branches back to within one to two pairs of leaves above where the stems become woody.
Drying: Hang stems upside down to air dry.

USES

Cooking: Use fresh or dried sage leaves in stuffings and breads, with vegetables, tofu, or cheeses, and with many meats.
Oils: Use sage to flavor your favorite cooking oil.
Cosmetic: Add sage to infusions or oils to tone the skin. In rinses and conditioners, sage conditions dry hair and adds body. Deodorize feet with a soak in sage-scented water.
Crafts: Use dried sage leaves as the background for an herbal wreath.

Attention required

✓ Friendly to

✓ Ornamental

✓ Container growing

Yield

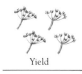
Easy to grow

Santolina

Santolina chamaecyparissus

Attention required

Friendly to ✗

Ornamental ✓

Container growing ✗

Yield

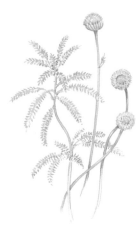

In perennial beds or herb gardens, the fine, lacy foliage of santolina adds a softening touch that lasts through the winter when the plants retain their leaves. The dried leaves are a staple of pest-repelling potpourris.

DESCRIPTION

Perennial
2 feet tall
Zones 6 to 8
Flowers: Clusters of yellow buttonlike flowers bloom in midsummer.
Leaves: The narrow alternate leaves are silvery or grayish green.
Flavor and fragrance: Strong, lavender-like fragrance.

HOW TO GROW

When to plant: Plant seeds indoors eight weeks before your last spring frost date. Wait until all danger of frost has passed to transplant the seedlings to the garden. Or sow seeds directly in the garden one week before the last spring frost date. Layer stems in early spring; divide plants in spring or fall; or take cuttings in spring and early summer.
Where to plant: Prefers full sun.
Soil and fertility: Plant santolina in well-drained soil of low to moderate fertility and with a pH of 6.5 to 7.5. Allow

the top inch of soil to dry between waterings.
Plant spacing: Allow 1 to 2 feet between plants.
Pests: Usually pest-free
Diseases: Susceptible to root rot in soggy soils

HARVESTING

When to harvest: Harvest leafy branches in midsummer. If harvesting for flowers, wait until blooms begin to open. Gather flowers in the morning after the dew has dried. For most successful drying, harvest

during dry weather.
How to harvest: Cut whole stems 3 to 4 inches above the soil surface. Cut flowers with long stems for easier drying and greater versatility in dried arrangements.
Drying: Hang stems with leaves or flowers to air dry.

USES

Arrangements and crafts: Use santolina branches as base material for herbal wreaths. The dried flowers add wonderful yellow accents to winter bouquets and potpourris.
Insect repellent: Santolina is one of the most effective insect-repelling herbs. Use it in lotions, potpourris, and sachets.

TIPS

Because of its fragrance, santolina is also called lavender cotton. However, it is from the aster family.

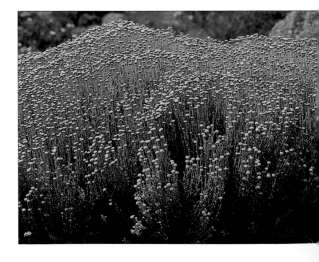

▶ **Santolina** *can make a stunning display plant on its own or in combination with other herbs. Try growing it behind some lemon or silver thyme for contrast.*

Savory, summer

Satureja hortensis

The slender stems and small leaves of summer savory are pretty enough to tuck into flower arrangements for the table where you can enjoy their wonderful fragrance.

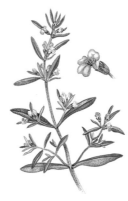

DESCRIPTION
Annual
18 inches tall
Flowers: White or pale pink, ¼-inch-long flowers bloom in groups of three to six at upper leaf axils (where the leaves join the stems) from midsummer until frost.
Leaves: The smooth gray-green 1-inch-long leaves are narrow and opposite.
Flavor and fragrance: Summer savory has a peppery flavor and aroma that's somewhat milder than that of winter savory.

HOW TO GROW
When to plant: Sow seeds directly in the garden a week before your last spring frost date. Or start seeds indoors six weeks before your last spring frost date, and transplant seedlings to the garden after all danger of frost has passed.
Where to plant: Prefers full sun.
Soil and fertility: Plant in well-drained soil of average fertility and keep it moderately moist. A pH of 6.8 to 7.0 is ideal.

Plant spacing: Space plants 10 inches apart.
Pests: Usually pest-free
Diseases: Susceptible to leaf spot and other fungal diseases if humidity is too high. Plant where air circulation is good and do not crowd.

HARVESTING
When to harvest: Pick small sprigs anytime after the plant reaches a height of 6 to 8 inches. Harvest stems for drying before the plant flowers. Harvest in the morning after the dew dries.
How to harvest: Cut off stem tips when harvesting small amounts; this will also delay flowering. For drying, cut whole stems several inches above the soil surface.
Drying: Hang stems upside down to air dry, or dry them on screens.
Freezing: Freeze in butter or ice cubes.

USES
Cooking: Use fresh or dried summer savory leaves to season beans of all kinds. This herb is also good with cheeses, eggs, cabbage-family crops, parsnips, squash, chicken, fish, and in soups, sauces, and marinades.
Vinegars: Use in vinegars for a light, delicious flavor.
Medicinal: A strong infusion of summer savory aids digestion.
Crafts: Add the dried leaves to potpourris.

TIPS
Summer savory makes a wonderful container plant because of the graceful, drooping habit of its stems. For winter production, start seeds in August or September and grow them inside under a plant light through the winter.

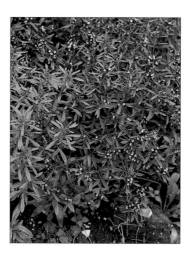

▲ **Summer savory** *is one of the prettiest annual herbs you can grow.*

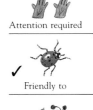
Attention required

✓ Friendly to

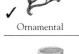
✓ Ornamental

✓ Container growing

Yield

Easy to grow

Savory, winter

Satureja montana

The often-evergreen leaves of winter savory can help to keep the memories of your herb garden alive during the winter months. In spring, it's one of the first fragrances you'll enjoy.

Attention required

Friendly to ✓

Ornamental ✓

Container growing ✓

Yield

Easy to grow

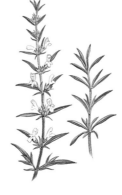

DESCRIPTION
Perennial
16 inches tall
Zones 5 to 10
Flowers: Spikes of small white to purplish flowers bloom atop the plants in early summer.
Leaves: The narrowly oval, opposite, 1-inch-long leaves have smooth edges and are wider at the tip end than at the base. Winter savory is semi-evergreen in moderate climates or in protected sites.
Flavor and fragrance: Winter savory has a strong, sharp peppery flavor and aroma.

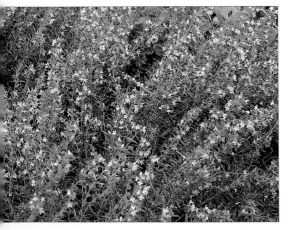

HOW TO GROW
When to plant: Buy young plants and transplant them to your garden in spring or summer. Or sow seeds indoors eight to ten weeks before your last spring frost date. Transplant seedlings to the garden after all danger of frost has passed. Cuttings root easily. Take them in spring when the plant has resumed rapid growth.
Where to plant: Prefers full sun but will tolerate filtered shade.
Soil and fertility: Plant in well-drained light soil of low to moderate fertility. Do not apply compost more than once every two years; high nitrogen levels make winter savory more susceptible to diseases.
Plant spacing: Space plants 1 foot apart.
Pests: Usually pest-free
Diseases: Susceptible to root rot and winterkill in soggy soils

◄ **Winter savory** *may be pruned into a small hedge for formal gardens.*

HARVESTING
When to harvest: Harvest small sprigs as needed. For drying, harvest before or after the plant blooms. For best quality, gather leafy stems in the morning after the dew dries.
How to harvest: Snip off branch tips for small amounts. When harvesting larger quantities for drying, cut whole stems to about 6 inches above the soil surface; cut again near the end of the summer.
Drying: Hang stems upside down to air dry.

USES
Cooking: This strongly flavored herb is best used in crab dishes and with other strong flavors. It overpowers chicken but is just right in pâtés and meat pies.
Vinegars: Use winter savory in vinegars for an interesting flavor.

CULTIVARS AND RELATIVES
● Dwarf winter savory (*S. montana* 'Nana'): Use this 3- to 4-inch-tall cultivar to edge your herb garden or perennial border.

TIPS
Older plants become rangy and untidy. Lightly prune winter savory in late winter to keep it compact and neat looking.

Southernwood

Artemisia abrotanum

The gray-green leaves and upright growth of southernwood make it an outstanding focal point in a garden or even in a foundation planting around your house. Just brushing the leaves releases their clean fragrance.

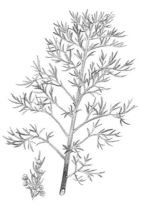

DESCRIPTION
Perennial
To 5 feet tall
Zones 4 to 8
Flowers: Loose clusters of tiny, inconspicuous greenish-yellowish-white flowers bloom in late summer. Southernwood rarely blooms in northern areas.
Leaves: Fine, feathery, downy, gray-green leaves cover stems that become woody as the plant ages. In mild areas, plants hold their leaves through the winter.
Flavor and fragrance: Southernwood is not typically recommended for internal use; it has a strong, clean, almost camphorlike fragrance.

HOW TO GROW
When to plant: Buy young plants and transplant them to the garden in spring or summer. Take cuttings in early summer or divide established plants in spring.
Where to plant: Prefers full sun.
Soil and fertility: Plant in well-drained soil of average fertility. Apply $\frac{1}{2}$ inch of compost as a mulch every spring. Allow the top 1 to 2 inches of soil to dry between waterings.
Plant spacing: Space plants 2 to 4 feet apart.
Pests: Pest-free
Diseases: Susceptible to root rot in poorly drained soils

HARVESTING
When to harvest: Harvest stems anytime. For best drying, gather stems in the morning after the dew dries.
How to harvest: Cut whole stems back to the woody portions.
Drying: Hang stems upside down to air dry.

USES
Medicinal: A decoction of southernwood branches and barley is said to be effective against acne.
Cosmetic: Use southernwood leaves and bark in hair rinses and conditioners to condition oily hair, help prevent dandruff, and give hair body.
Arrangements and crafts: Use dried southernwood branches as a base for herbal wreaths. Add dried stems to winter arrangements or use fresh branches in summer bouquets.
Insect repellent: Southernwood is an excellent insect repellent. Use it in insect-repelling sachets and lotions, and keep branches in linen closets.

Attention required

Friendly to

Ornamental

Container growing

Yield

Easy to grow

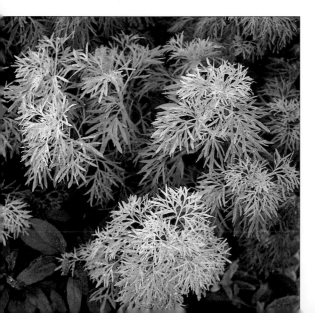

◀ **Southern-wood's** *distinctive form and gray-green color make it an excellent focal point for your herb garden.*

Sweet cicely

Myrrhis odorata

The ferny stems and tiny white flowers of sweet cicely are a pretty backdrop in the shade garden, where they'll naturalize nicely, giving you plenty of licorice-flavored roots, seeds, and leaves for cooking and baking.

Attention required

Friendly to ✓

Ornamental ✓

Container growing ✗

Yield

Easy to grow

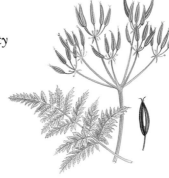

DESCRIPTION
Perennial
To 3 feet tall
Zones 3 to 7
Flowers: Queen-Anne's-lace-like umbels of tiny white flowers bloom in May or June.
Leaves: Ferny, finely lobed or toothed leaflets are clear green with whitish undersides. The leafstalks wrap around the stem of the plant. Plants die back in the winter.
Flavor and fragrance: Sweet cicely has a very sweet flavor with a hint of licorice; its fragrance is like that of lovage.

HOW TO GROW
When to plant: Buy young plants and transplant them to the garden in spring or summer. Seeds germinate only after undergoing a series of freezes and thaws. Fresh seed planted in the late summer or early fall may or may not germinate. Divide sweet cicely in spring to early summer by digging down to look for buds on the roots. Carefully cut through the root mass to take a piece of the rootstock with a bud on it. Pat the soil back around the remaining roots and plant the new plant at the same depth at which it was growing.
Where to plant: Prefers shade or partial shade; dies easily in full sun.
Soil and fertility: Plant in rich, moist, well-drained soil. Apply ½ inch of compost every spring.
Plant spacing: Space plants 2 feet apart.
Pests: Usually pest-free
Diseases: Usually disease-free

HARVESTING
When to harvest: Pick sweet cicely leaves anytime. Harvest seeds on a midsummer afternoon when they are ripe and dry. Dig roots after they are a year old.
How to harvest: Snip off leaves whenever needed. For drying, cut whole stems. Enclose seed heads before seeds begin to brown and cut them with a length of stem just as they begin to shatter. Dig roots with a spading fork.
Drying: Hang stems upside down to dry leaves or bagged seed heads.
Freezing: Freeze leaves in oil or ice cubes.

USES
Cooking: Use fresh leaves in salads and with fruits. The dried or frozen leaves are excellent with fish. Use seeds in cakes and desserts. Cook fresh or dried roots as a parsniplike vegetable or add them to soups and stews.

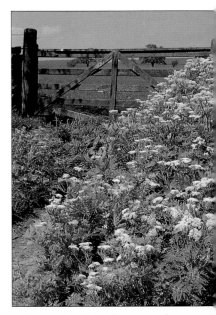

▲ **Sweet cicely** *self-sows with ease.*

TIPS
If you use sweet cicely seeds in baked goods, you can decrease the sugar in the recipe.

Sweet woodruff

Galium odoratum

A lush spread of sweet woodruff makes a beautiful groundcover in the shady areas under trees. Violets and early-flowering Japanese iris set off its lovely white blooms.

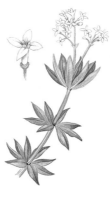

DESCRIPTION
Perennial
8 to 12 inches tall
Zones 3 to 9
Flowers: Showy white clusters of small, funnel-shaped, four-petaled blossoms appear in loose clusters above the foliage in spring.
Leaves: Interesting whorls of six to eight lance-shaped bright green leaves grow directly from the stems.
Flavor and fragrance: No longer recommended for internal use, sweet woodruff has the clean fresh aroma of newly mowed hay. As it dries, the foliage develops a vanilla scent.

HOW TO GROW
When to plant: Buy young plants and transplant them to the garden in spring or summer. The seeds are notorious for being difficult to germinate. Sow seeds in the fall where they are to grow, and let them freeze and thaw over the winter. Germination is apt to be spotty, so plant thickly. Some seeds will wait a year to sprout. Once sweet woodruff is firmly established, it will self-sow if it likes the site. Divide established plants in the very early spring.
Where to plant: Prefers shade but tolerates partial shade.
Soil and fertility: Plant in moist, humus-rich soil with a pH of 5.0 to 5.5. If you grow sweet woodruff under hardwood trees, leave the leaf litter in place and it will adequately feed the plants over the years. Plants without this source of nutrition require yearly applications of ½ to 1 inch of compost in late winter.
Plant spacing: Space plants 8 inches apart.

Pests: Usually pest-free
Diseases: Usually disease-free

HARVESTING
When to harvest: Harvest leaves anytime once plants are established.
How to harvest: Snip leaves with stems.
Drying: Hang stems upside down to air dry.

USES
Arrangements and crafts: Add dried sweet woodruff to potpourris, sachets, and herbal wreaths.

TIPS
Sweet woodruff is traditionally used to add a vanilla-like flavor to wines and other alcoholic beverages. The U.S. Food and Drug Administration considers these uses to be safe but warns against eating sweet woodruff because of the risk of damage to the liver and other organs. Place potpourris containing sweet woodruff where children cannot reach them.

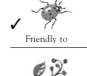
Attention required

✓ Friendly to

✓ Ornamental

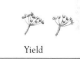
✗ Container growing

Yield

Easy to grow

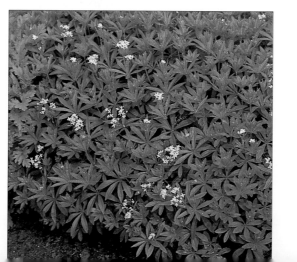

◄ **Sweet woodruff** *provides a graceful reminder that spring has arrived in wooded areas.*

Tansy

Tanacetum vulgare

Sunny yellow tansy flowers make a strong display in the garden or dried in winter bouquets. In addition, these long-lived plants will give you plenty of leaves for insect-repelling lotions.

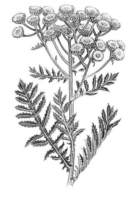

Attention required

 ✗
Friendly to

 ✓
Ornamental

✓
Container growing

Yield

Easy to grow

DESCRIPTION
Perennial
3 to 4 feet tall
Zones 4 to 8
Flowers: Bright yellow clusters of many small buttonlike flowers bloom at the tops of the stems from midsummer until early fall.
Leaves: The ferny leaves are divided into about 12 leaflets with toothed edges. Plants die back in winter.
Flavor and fragrance: Tansy is not recommended for internal use; it has a strong, somewhat bitter aroma.

HOW TO GROW
When to plant: Plant seeds indoors six to eight weeks before your last spring frost date, and transplant seedlings to the garden after all danger of frost has passed. Divide established plants in spring or fall.
Where to plant: Prefers partial or filtered shade but will tolerate full sun if soil is moist.
Soil and fertility: Plant tansy in moist well-drained soil of average fertility. Plants need about an inch of moisture every week. Apply ½ inch of compost every spring.
Plant spacing: Allow 3 to 4 feet between plants.
Pests: Aphids
Diseases: Usually disease-free

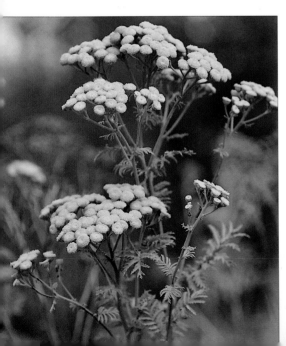

◄ **Tansy** *is such a useful companion plant that gardeners sometimes hesitate to pull out all the volunteers it produces. But it's prolific enough to become weedy.*

HARVESTING
When to harvest: Harvest tansy leaves anytime. For best quality, harvest in the morning after the dew dries. Pick flowers in the afternoon from midsummer to fall when they are almost fully open.
How to harvest: Cut whole stems, with or without flowers.
Drying: Hang stems upside down to air dry.

USES
Cooking: Don't use tansy in cooking, even though you may find recipes in older herbals that include it. This plant may cause illness when taken internally.
Medicinal: Extract the active ingredients in tansy in a light oil to make a skin lotion that helps to control acne.
Arrangements: Fresh-cut tansy flowers are a nice addition to a summer bouquet. Stems of dried flowers add a tall, colorful note to arrangements.
Insect repellent: Tansy repels many insects. Keep pots of it near all your doors to discourage ants from entering. Use it in insect-repelling lotions. Include the dried leaves and flowers in pest-repellent cushions for your pets.

TIPS
Tansy self-sows abundantly. Fortunately, it's easy to pull, so you shouldn't let this stop you from growing it.

Tarragon, French

Artemisia dracunculus var. *sativa*

*Tarragon adds sophistication –
both to your cooking and to the herb
garden. The leafy stems are beautiful
in herb vinegars and the resulting
flavor is a wonderful addition to
poultry dishes.*

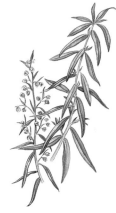

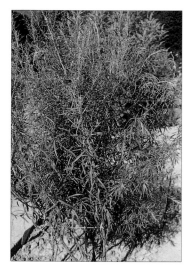

▲ **French tarragon** *is one of
the first herbs to come up in
spring.*

DESCRIPTION

Perennial
To 2 feet tall
Zones 4 to 8
Flowers: Tiny, round,
inconspicuous flowers bloom at
the stem tips in midsummer.
Leaves: The narrow,
smooth-edged leaves are 1 to 4
inches long. They grow in
groups of three at the base of
the plant and singly at the top.
Plants die back in winter.
Flavor and fragrance: Tarragon
has a sweet, aniselike flavor
with a bit of a bite; its
fragrance is similar.

HOW TO GROW

When to plant: Buy a young
plant and transplant it to the
garden in spring or summer.
Tarragon seeds are generally
sterile. Take a nibble of a leaf
before purchasing to make sure
it has a fresh licorice flavor.
Take cuttings from year-old
plants in the fall and
overwinter them indoors until
the following spring, or divide
plants in early spring after they
are three years old.
Where to plant: Prefers full
sun; tolerates filtered shade.
Soil and fertility: Plant in
well-drained fertile soil. Apply
½ inch of compost in the early
spring each year.
Plant spacing: Allow 2 square
feet per plant.
Pests: Usually pest-free
Diseases: Susceptible to root
rot in poorly drained soil; may
develop downy mildew or
powdery mildew in crowded
conditions.

HARVESTING

When to harvest: Pick tarragon
leaves anytime. For best flavor,
gather them in the morning.
How to harvest: Snip off
branch tips. For drying, cut
whole branches. Cut back in
June to stimulate new growth.
Drying: Use a dehydrator;
tarragon loses quality unless
rapidly dried.
Freezing: Freezing captures the
flavor better than drying. Freeze
in oils, butter, or ice cubes.

USES

Cooking: Use fresh tarragon in
salads (sparingly – it's strong)
and in sauces. Use it in meat or
poultry dishes. With the
exception of recipes that are
baked in liquid, such as chicken
in white wine, add the tarragon
at the very end of the cooking
time to avoid bringing out a
bitter taste.
Vinegars: Tarragon gives
an unusual licorice flavor.
Oils: You can flavor cooking
oils with tarragon, but it's more
commonly added to vinegars.

TIPS

The seeds of Russian tarragon
(*A. dracunculus*) are often
passed off as "tarragon" seeds.
This plant lacks the flavor of
French tarragon.

Attention required

✗ Friendly to

✓ Ornamental

✓ Container growing

Yield

Easy to grow

Thyme

Thymus spp.

Attention required

Friendly to ✓

Ornamental ✓

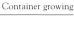
Container growing ✓

Yield

Easy to grow

A garden of thymes with all their wonderful fragrances, colors, and leaf forms is a delight to the senses. Plant a sampler of your favorite cultivars. These durable, spreading plants make attractive groundcovers along a path.

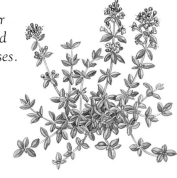

DESCRIPTION

Perennial
6 to 15 inches tall, depending on species and cultivar
Zones 5 to 9
Flowers: Clusters of tiny pink to purple tubular blooms at the stem tips in midsummer.
Leaves: Most of the thymes have small, narrow, $\frac{1}{4}$- to $\frac{1}{2}$-inch-long leaves with pale, hairy undersides and smooth edges. Stems become woody with age and may retain leaves through the winter months.
Flavor and fragrance: Most cultivars have a strong, slightly sharp flavor and aroma.

HOW TO GROW

When to plant: Sow five to eight seeds per pot, eight to ten weeks before your last spring frost date. Transplant seedlings to the garden a week before that date. Many cultivars do not come true from seed; buy these as plants. Layer stems in late spring to early summer, take cuttings in spring, and divide plants in spring or fall.
Where to plant: Prefers full sun but tolerates partial shade.
Soil and fertility: Plant in well-drained light soil of low to moderate fertility. Excess nitrogen increases susceptibility to fungal diseases.
Plant spacing: Allow 1 foot between groups of plants.
Pests: Spider mites
Diseases: Root rot, leaf spot

HARVESTING

When to harvest: Harvest leaves in the morning whenever plants are not in bloom.
How to harvest: Snip off stem tips. When collecting larger quantities for drying, cut the entire plant back to 2 inches above the soil just before it blooms. Take only branch tips for the rest of the season.
Drying: Enclose bunched stems upside down in paper sacks and hang to air dry. Or place stems on the fruit leather insert of a dehydrator.
Freezing: Freeze sprigs of thyme on a baking sheet and then store them in an airtight freezer container. Freeze in butter or ice cubes.

USES

Cooking: Thyme goes with almost everything. Fresh leaves are a nice addition to a salad. Try it fresh or dried with seafood, poultry, vegetables, legumes, cheese, eggs, rice, and tomato sauces. Frozen sprigs are handy for soups or stews.
Oils: Use thyme to flavor your favorite cooking oil.
Medicinal: An infusion of thyme settles the stomach.
Cosmetic: Add thyme to bathwater for a refreshing bath. It has antiseptic qualities that make it especially good for raw, rough skin.
Crafts: Add thyme to potpourris for a clean, almost piney scent.
Insect repellent: Use thyme in a potpourri for repelling insects.

▼ **Thyme** *makes a pretty groundcover.*

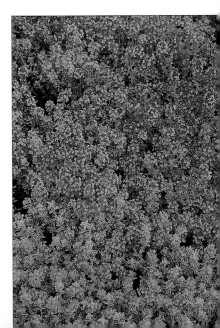

Valerian

Valeriana officinalis

Valerian is also called garden heliotrope – under this name it is known as an old-time flower bed favorite for its colorful and fragrant blossoms. Its aroma was once considered worthy of adding to cosmetics.

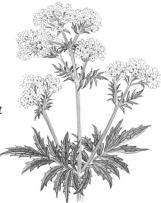

DESCRIPTION
Perennial
To 5 feet tall
Zones 4 to 7
Flowers: Large clusters, up to 4 inches across, of small pink to purple tubular flowers bloom in early June.
Leaves: Opposite pairs of leaves are deeply lobed or divided on short stems from the main branches. A terminal leaflet grows on each leaf stem. Hairs grow along the veins on the undersides of the leaves. Plants die back over winter.
Flavor and fragrance: Valerian has a very bitter flavor. Its fragrance is strong and clean with a musty undertone.

HOW TO GROW
When to plant: Buy young plants and transplant them to the garden in spring. Plant seeds in the garden one to two weeks before your last spring frost date. Or start seeds early indoors, eight weeks before your last spring frost date, in peat or newspaper pots. Put several seeds in each pot and plant more pots than you need. Transplant to the garden after all danger of frost has passed. Plants spread by runners; propagate by digging and transplanting them once the mother plant is established. Divide mature plants in spring.
Where to plant: Prefers full sun but tolerates partial or filtered shade.
Soil and fertility: Plant in rich, moist, well-drained soil. Apply ½ inch of compost every spring.
Plant spacing: Allow 1 foot between plants.
Pests: Usually pest-free
Diseases: Usually disease-free

HARVESTING
When to harvest: Harvest valerian roots in the fall.
How to harvest: Dig roots with a spading fork after five days or more of dry weather.
Drying: Cut the roots into 1- to 2-inch pieces and dry them on screens or in a dehydrator.

USES
Medicinal: Valerian contains a potent active ingredient that has a sedative effect; it is used as a tranquilizer in concentrated doses. Use it with caution and only for limited periods of time – extended use can cause depression. For home use, an infusion of the roots makes a calming, sleep-promoting tea; add honey to make it palatable. Because the amount of active ingredient in a home preparation is variable, do not give valerian tea to children.
Cosmetic: Add valerian root to your bathwater for a calming soak before bed.

TIPS
Cats like the smell of valerian, so use it in an insect-repelling pillow for your pet.

Attention required

✓ Friendly to

✓ Ornamental

✓ Container growing

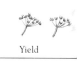
Yield

Easy to grow

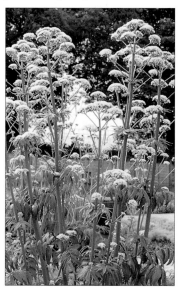

▲ **Valerian** *needs to be divided regularly.*

Vervain, European

Verbena officinalis

The wonderful fragrance of vervain makes it a delightful addition to your bath. Cats like its scent almost as much as the aroma of catnip, and respond to it with pleasure.

Attention required

Friendly to ✓

Ornamental ✓

Container growing ✓

Yield

Easy to grow

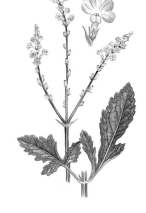

DESCRIPTION
Annual
3 feet tall
Flowers: Tall spikes of tiny purplish white tubular flowers bloom at the top of the plant in spring.
Leaves: The narrow leaves are opposite with toothed edges.
Flavor and fragrance: European vervain is not recommended for internal use; it has a fresh, green scent that is somewhat calming.

HOW TO GROW
When to plant: Sow seeds in the garden about two weeks before your last spring frost date. Or take cuttings from the new growth of overwintered plants.
Where to plant: Prefers full sun.
Soil and fertility: Plant in rich, well-drained but moist soil.
Plant spacing: Space plants 1 foot apart.
Pests: Usually pest-free
Diseases: Usually disease-free

HARVESTING
When to harvest: Harvest leaves and stems anytime. For best quality, gather in the morning after the dew dries.
How to harvest: Cut whole stems.
Drying: Hang stems upside down to air dry.

USES
Cosmetic: Add vervain to your bathwater for a soothing bath.

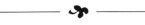

CULTIVARS AND RELATIVES
- Blue vervain (*V. hastata*): A common wildflower that grows in damp areas. It looks very much like European vervain, except that its flowers are more purple-blue.

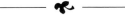

TIPS
Older herbals recommend drinking a tea made from vervain; however, contemporary researchers report that this tea causes vomiting, even at low strengths.

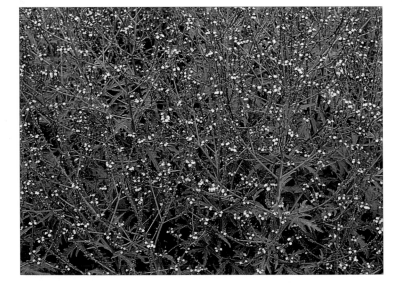

◀ **European vervain** *gives a graceful, airy look to any garden. Be sure to harvest some stems before they flower if you want to use them in the bath.*

Violet

Viola odorata

The charm of violets never fades. While today we enjoy them in salads or crystallized on cakes, to the Greeks they represented fertility and the Romans used them as a cure for insomnia.

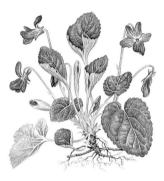

DESCRIPTION

Perennial
To 6 inches tall
Zones 5 to 8

Flowers: Purple, blue, pink, or white ½-inch flowers have two upper petals and three below; the central bottom petal forms a tube at the base that contains the anthers. The petals are often streaked or striped. Violets bloom in early spring.

Leaves: Oval, kidney- or heart-shaped, dark green leaves are smooth or downy and reach 2½ inches wide. Plants die back in winter.

Flavor and fragrance: Violet flowers have a delicate sweet flavor and aroma.

HOW TO GROW

When to plant: Buy young plants and transplant them to the garden in spring, summer, or early fall. Plant seeds in the fall where they are to grow so they can experience the many freeze-thaw periods they need for germination. If you plant seeds in the spring, simulate these conditions by freezing the seed for two weeks, letting it thaw for a day or two, refreezing, and thawing again. Plant it in the garden as soon as you can scratch a furrow in the soil. Divide established plants in early spring, just as their leaves begin to peek above the soil.

Where to plant: Prefers partial shade but tolerates full sun.

Soil and fertility: Plant violets in moist but well-drained, rich soil. Mulch each fall with chopped hardwood leaves for winter protection and a source of nutrients through the season.

Plant spacing: Space plants 1 foot apart.

Pests: Slugs, spider mites

Diseases: Crown rot, downy mildew, leaf spot

HARVESTING

When to harvest: Pick flowers when they are fully open. Gather young leaves in early spring.

How to harvest: Cut each flower or leaf with its stem.

Drying: Press between sheets of absorbent paper placed inside a book. Store dried flowers in complete darkness for best color retention.

Crystallizing: Crystallize fresh flowers.

USES

Cooking: Fresh flowers are an excellent edible garnish. Float them on fruit soups and punches. Add them to fruit salads, green salads, and gelatins. Use crystallized flowers to decorate cakes, pies, and pastries. Add the young leaves to salads.

Crafts: Violets can be added to potpourris, but they lose fragrance quickly and their color fades in sunlight.

▼ **Violets** *spread so rapidly that you'll never be without them once your first plants become established.*

Attention required

✓ Friendly to

✓ Ornamental

✓ Container growing

Yield

Easy to grow

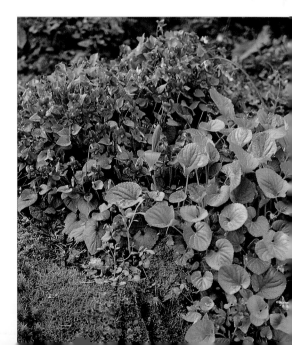

Wormwood

Artemisia absinthium

Wormwood is a plant of striking appearance, particularly in the winter when its angular branches stand out against the starkness of the landscape. Its strong, musky fragrance delights the noses of some, while others find it less pleasant.

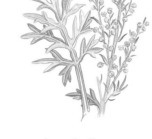

Attention required

 ✗
Friendly to

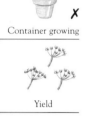 ✓
Ornamental

 ✗
Container growing

Yield

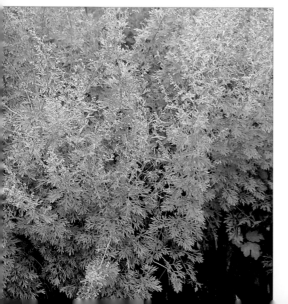
Easy to grow

DESCRIPTION

Perennial

4 feet tall

Zones 4 to 6

Flowers: Clusters of small yellowish green round flowers bloom in midsummer.

Leaves: The ferny gray-green leaves are deeply divided and covered with soft, fine hairs. Plants become woody with age.

Flavor and fragrance: Although its history includes a variety of internal uses, wormwood is no longer considered safe to eat. It has a pungent, bitter aroma that smells wonderfully clean to some people and offensive to others.

HOW TO GROW

When to plant: Plant wormwood seeds indoors ten weeks before your last spring frost date, and transplant seedlings to the garden a week before that date. Or sow seeds directly in the garden in fall. Take cuttings in early spring; divide plants in spring or fall.

Where to plant: Prefers full sun but tolerates partial shade.

Soil and fertility: Plant in well-drained soil of low to moderate fertility. Apply compost once every three years.

Plant spacing: Allow 3 feet between plants and between wormwood and other plants.

Pests: Pest-free

Diseases: Usually disease-free

◀ **Wormwood** *makes an outstanding background plant.*

HARVESTING

When to harvest: Harvest branches when the plants are in bloom in midsummer.

How to harvest: Cut off only the tops of branches with a sharp pair of pruners. Vigorous plants will withstand two harvests in a growing season.

Drying: Hang branches upside down to air dry.

USES

Arrangements and crafts: Use the dried flowers in winter bouquets and wreaths; add dried leaves to sachets. Wormwood's gray-green foliage makes a nice accent in a fresh bouquet.

Insect repellent: Add to homemade insect repellents.

CULTIVARS AND RELATIVES

- 'Silver King' (*A. ludoviciana* 'Silver King'): Lovely white flowers top stems of silver-white leaves.
- Sweet wormwood, annual wormwood (*A. annua*): This is a delight in the garden or in dried wreaths and winter bouquets. Strong, fruity fragrance.

TIPS

Wormwood lives about seven years and is most productive in its second and third years. If you want large harvests every year, plant successively, starting a new plant or two every year.

Yarrow

Achillea millefolium

This herb gets its botanical name from Achilles, who was said to have used the mashed leaves as a poultice to stanch the bleeding from wounds. Try it on the next scraped knee at your house – your children will be delighted.

DESCRIPTION

Perennial
1 to 3 feet tall, depending on species and cultivar
Zones 2 to 8
Flowers: Flattened clusters of small flowers, in colors ranging from white to yellow, pink, and purple, bloom in midsummer through fall.
Leaves: The ferny divided leaves are about 1 inch wide and 6 inches long.
Flavor and fragrance: Yarrow may cause allergic reactions when taken internally. It has a pleasantly bitter aroma.

HOW TO GROW

When to plant: Plant seeds in the garden a week before your last spring frost date. Or start them indoors, in plantable pots of peat or newspaper, eight weeks before your last spring frost date. Transplant seedlings to the garden after all danger of frost has passed. Divide plants in early spring.
Where to plant: Prefers full sun but tolerates partial shade.
Soil and fertility: Plant in well-drained moderately fertile soil. Yarrow grows well in a variety of soil types and fertility levels. For more flowers, add ½ inch of compost around plants every spring.
Plant spacing: Space plants 1 foot apart.
Pests: Usually pest-free
Diseases: Powdery mildew, rust, stem rot

HARVESTING

When to harvest: Harvest flowers from summer to fall when they are fully open, but before the flower heads have begun to curl downward. Gather them in the morning after the dew dries.
How to harvest: Cut whole stems. Prolong the bloom period by removing all flowers before they set seed.
Drying: Strip off the leaves and hang stems upside down to air dry. Yarrow flowers hold their colors well when dried.

USES

Cosmetic: Use yarrow in skin lotions for its astringent qualities. In hair rinses and conditioners, yarrow leaves and flowers condition oily hair.
Arrangements: Use fresh or dried flowers to add color.

Attention required

✓ Friendly to

✓ Ornamental

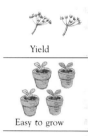
✓ Container growing

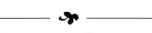
Yield

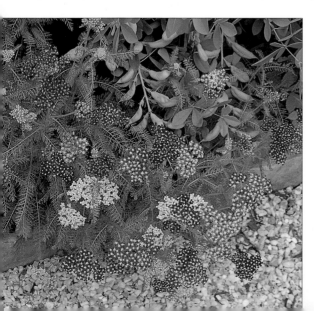

◀ **Yarrow** *flowers attract beneficials, including the tiny wasps that feed on aphids. Plant some near your fruit and vegetable gardens.*

Easy to grow

CULTIVARS AND RELATIVES

● Garden mace (*A. decolorans*): The fragrance of this yarrow resembles true mace; some people add the leaves of this species to salads.

USDA Plant Hardiness Zone Map

This map was revised in 1990 to reflect changes in climate since the original USDA map, done in 1965. It is now recognized as the best estimator of minimum temperatures available. Look at the map to find your area, then match its pattern to the key on the right. When you've found your pattern, the key will tell you what hardiness zone you live in. Remember that the map is a general guide; your particular conditions may vary.

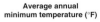

Average annual minimum temperature (°F)

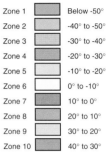

Zone 1	Below -50°
Zone 2	-40° to -50°
Zone 3	-30° to -40°
Zone 4	-20° to -30°
Zone 5	-10° to -20°
Zone 6	0° to -10°
Zone 7	10° to 0°
Zone 8	20° to 10°
Zone 9	30° to 20°
Zone 10	40° to 30°

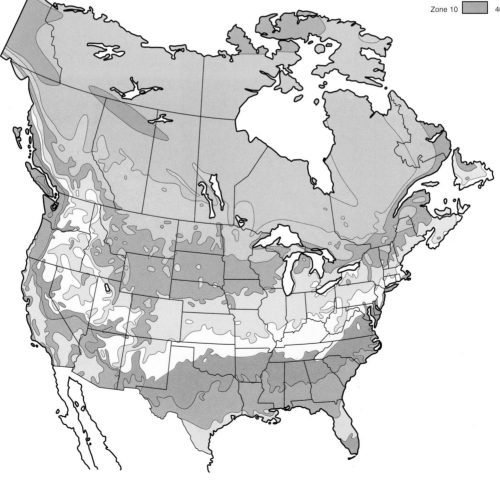

Resources

HERB ASSOCIATIONS
The Herb Growers and
Marketing Network
P.O. Box 245
Silver Spring, PA 17575
717-393-3295
fax 717-393-9261

Each year this association of
amateur and professional herb
growers and suppliers prints *The
Herbal Green Pages*, a 300+
page listing of growers and
suppliers, as well as four large
newsletters that report research
and information about all
aspects of the herb business.

SEED AND PLANT SUPPLIERS
Bountiful Gardens
18001 Shafer Ranch Rd.
Willits, CA 95490-9626
707-459-6410
*Organically grown and
open-pollinated herb and vegetable
seeds, gardening supplies*

Capriland's Herb Farm
534 Silver St.
Coventry, CT 06238
203-742-7244
*More than 300 varieties of herb
plants and seeds, wreaths, dolls,
tours, lectures, gardens*

Companion Plants
7247 N. Coolville Ridge Rd.
Athens, OH 45701
614-592-4643
*Herbs for all uses – aromatic,
culinary, dye, ornamental,
repellents*

The Cook's Garden
P.O. Box 535
Londonderry, VT 05148
802-824-3400
*Culinary vegetable and herb seeds,
books, garden supplies*

The Gourmet Gardener
8650 College Blvd.
Overland Park, KS 66210
913-345-0490
fax 913-451-2443
Herb seeds, books

Le Jardin du Gourmet
P.O. Box 75, Memorial Dr.
St. Johnsbury Center, VT 05863
802-748-1446
fax 802-748-9592
Herb seeds

Nichols Garden Nursery
1190 N. Pacific Hwy.
Albany, OR 97321-4580
541-928-9280
*Herb seeds and plants, garlic and
shallot bulbs, books, spices,
potpourris, teas, accessories,
garden supplies*

Richters
Goodwood
Ontario, Canada L0C 1A0
905-640-6677
fax 905-640-6641
Internet:
  orderdesk@richters.com
  custserv@richters.com
  info@richters.com
  http://www.richters.com
*Herb plants and seeds, garden
supplies*

Sandy Mush Herb Nursery
316 Surrett Cove Rd.
Leicester, NC 28748
704-683-2014
*More than 600 culinary, tea,
decorative, and scented herbs,
scented geraniums, dye plants,
flowering perennials, seeds,
topiary plants and frames, recipes,
books, gourmet vegetables*

Shepherd's Garden Seeds
30 Irene St.
Torrington, CT 06790
860-482-3638
fax 860-482-0532
Herb seeds, garden supplies

Well-Sweep Herb Farm
205 Mt. Bethel Rd.
Port Murray, NJ 07865
908-852-5390
*Herb seeds and plants, books,
garden supplies, tours, lectures,
gardens*

SOIL-TESTING LABORATORIES
A&L Agricultural Laboratories
7621 Whitepine Rd.
Richmond, VA 23237

Cook's Consulting
R.D. 2, Box 13
Lowville, NY 13367

I.F.M.
333 Ohme Garden Rd.
Wenatchee, WA 98801

Woods End Agricultural
Institute, Old Rome Rd.
P.O. Box 297
Mt. Vernon, ME 04352

Recommended Reading

Carr, Anna, et al. *Rodale's Illustrated Encyclopedia of Herbs.* Edited by Claire Kowalchik and William H. Hylton. Emmaus, Pa.: Rodale Press, 1987.

Foster, Steven. *Herbal Renaissance: Growing, Using and Understanding Herbs in the Modern World.* Salt Lake City, Utah: Gibbs-Smith Publisher, 1993.

Gardner, Jo Ann. *The Heirloom Garden: Selecting & Growing Over 300 Old-Fashioned Ornamentals.* Pownal, Vt.: Storey Communications, 1992.

Grieve, Mrs. M. *A Modern Herbal.* New York: Dover Publications, 1971.

Hoffman, David. *The New Holistic Herbal.* Rockport, Mass.: Element Books, 1991.

Jeavons, John. *How to Grow More Vegetables Than You Ever Thought Possible on Less Land Than You Can Imagine.* 5th ed. Berkeley, Calif.: Ten Speed Press, 1995.

McClure, Susan. *The Herb Gardener.* Pownal, Vt.: Storey/Garden Way Publishing, 1996.

McHoy, Peter, and Pamela Westland. *The Herb Bible.* New York: Barnes and Noble, 1994.

Michalak, Patricia S. *Rodale's Successful Organic Gardening: Herbs.* Emmaus, Pa.: Rodale Press, 1993.

Oster, Maggie. *Herbal Vinegar.* Pownal, Vt.: Storey Publishing, 1994.

Reppert, Bertha. *Growing Your Herb Business.* Pownal, Vt.: Storey Publishing, 1994.

Rose, Jeanne. *Jeanne Rose's Modern Herbal.* New York: Perigee Books, Berkley Publishing Group, 1987.

Smith, Miranda, and Anna Carr. *Rodale's Garden Insect, Disease, and Weed Identification Guide.* Emmaus, Pa: Rodale Press, 1988.

Stella Natura, Kimberton Hills Agricultural Calendar, available from The Bio-Dynamic Farming and Gardening Association, Inc., PO Box 550, Kimberton, PA, 19442. 1-800-516-7797.

Tierra, Michael. *The Way of Herbs.* New York: Pocket Books, 1980.

Tyler, Varro E. *The Honest Herbal: A Sensible Guide to the Use of Herbs & Related Remedies.* 3rd ed. Binghamton, N.Y.: The Haworth Press, 1993.

Index